.

CHINESE HERBAL MEDICINE

CHINESE HERBAL MEDICINE

HOW TO USE
AND BENEFIT FROM
THE HEALING POWER
OF CHINESE HERBS

STEPHEN TANG ◆ RICHARD CRAZE

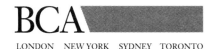

BCA

LONDON   NEW YORK   SYDNEY   TORONTO

Acknowledgements

The authors would like to thank the following people whose help and research have made this book possible: Ros Jay, Robert Miller of East West Herbs, and Susan Mears.

Chinese herbs should only be used under the guidance of a qualified Chinese herbalist. Neither the authors nor the publisher may be held responsible for any action or claim resulting from the use of this book or any information contained in it.

© Stephen Tang and Richard Craze

This edition published 1995
by BCA by arrangement with
Judy Piatkus (Publishers) Ltd

CN 4330

Printed in Great Britain

Contents

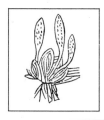

Caution

DIAGNOSIS AND TREATMENT

This is a book *about* Chinese herbal medicine, and is not primarily intended as a self-help handbook.

Self-diagnosis and treatment should only be used for the most minor of ailments, and a doctor should be consulted immediately if any symptoms persist or become aggravated. Symptoms such as high or low temperature, delirium or any other indication that the illness is more than a minor complaint should be reported to a doctor immediately.

Throughout this book you will find case histories of patients who have attended Stephen Tang's clinic in Manchester. Don't be tempted to correlate your symptoms and condition with those described, and to copy the medication provided. In Chinese herbal medicine every patient is unique, and what suits one person may not suit another.

In the hands of an experienced, qualified practitioner Chinese herbal medicine can sometimes be used to treat serious, even life-threatening, illnesses. But it should never be used in that way by anyone else.

Caution

Herbs

Many of the herbs referred to in this book are native to China, and are obtainable from reputable herbal stockists (see Useful Addresses). Don't confuse them with any similar-sounding, -looking or -tasting Western herbs; using another plant, even from the same family, will not produce the same results and may even be positively dangerous.

The herbs and prescriptions described in this book, when made up and used correctly, are not dangerous in themselves. However, certain combinations have great potency and must be handled and used with care.

Introduction

In the West when something happens
they ask what they can do about it.
In the East when something happens
we ask what has caused it.

Some people find their first acquaintance with Chinese medicine a little daunting, because it is so different from the conventional Western medicine to which they have been accustomed all their lives. The aim of this book is to make that first acquaintance a more friendly occasion, and to explain:

- how the various branches of Chinese medicine, in particular herbal medicine, work
- what conditions and illnesses it can best treat
- what Chinese herbalists are
- what their training comprises
- how they arrive at a diagnosis
- how they prescribe
- what effect herbal medicines may have
- what their long-term effects may be

Chinese medicine has evolved over thousands of years, and a good practitioner needs many years of experience. Some have been known to study and train for up to ten years, to spend twenty years practising, and then say that they are only just beginning to understand what it is all about. Co-author Stephen Tang, who can trace his ancestry back through thirty-six generations of Chinese herbalists, has himself been practising his art for over thirty years in the United Kingdom.

In the Chinese tradition, the whole approach to diagnosis and healing varies from the way in which Western doctors work. In the West, for instance, people seek cures when they have a problem, and expect the remedies to be as near instantaneous as possible. But the Chinese value the benefits of a more long-term approach: practitioners of herbal medicine also take into account lifestyle, diet, previous health conditions, any other medication which is being taken, and what type of person the patient is. They use their skills not only to treat existing complaints but also to prevent illness, to increase immunity and to enhance longevity.

The various branches of Chinese medicine are often used in an interconnecting way — acupuncture or massage, for example, may be given in conjunction with herbal remedies — whereas in the West each medical discipline is kept firmly separate from the others. Also, a course of treatment may take much longer than would harder-hitting, more aggressive Western medication, and the prescription may vary throughout the treatment. Frequently no specific illness is diagnosed; instead the symptoms are treated according to the fundamental concepts of Chinese philosophy — yin and yang, the Five Elements and qi (also commonly spelt ch'i in the West), to name but a few. Without some knowledge of these principles it would be impossible to understand anything of Chinese herbal medicine, for the underlying philosophy is as important as the herbal medication itself.

What we have attempted in this book is to weave a path through all these complexities and to explain the essentials as clearly as possible. It is intended not as a textbook but as an introductory guide for Western readers who may be undergoing, or thinking of undergoing, a course of herbal medicine, or who are interested in discovering more about this increasingly popular subject.

Let's start by stating as straightforwardly as possible the three main differences between Chinese herbal medicine and conventional Western treatments:

- Chinese herbal medicine treats *the whole person* rather than just the complaint – in other words, it is a form of holistic medicine.
- Chinese herbal medicine regards herbs as *benign* rather than as potions or poisons. (NB In the context of Chinese medicine 'herbs' means all plants, and not the limited Western interpretation which refers to food and cooking.)
- Chinese herbal medicine aims to *prevent illness* before it happens rather than cure it once it is present.

In today's climate of expanding awareness of alternative lifestyles and healthcare we are keen that Chinese herbal medicine should be more widely known and accepted in the West, because it has so much to offer people. We have seen for ourselves its ability both to heal those disorders that often fail to respond to the best of Western medicine, and to treat major diseases with methods that are more sympathetic to the human system and have fewer harmful side-effects.

Other authorities endorse this view. The World Health Organization has published a list of ailments and conditions for which treatment or alleviation with Chinese medicine is considered appropriate. They include:

- arthritis
- asthma
- cerebral palsy
- colitis
- depression
- diabetes

- eczema
- hay fever
- herpes
- hypoglycaemia
- impotence
- infertility
- insomnia
- pre-menstrual syndrome
- sciatica
- stroke
- vaginitis

Eminent Western doctors and scientists, too, are now making claims for plants which have been the stock-in-trade of Chinese herbalists for centuries. In the East the virtues of tea-drinking, for instance, have always been known, but more recently Professor Allan Conney of Rutgers University in New Jersey, USA, reported in the American journal *Cancer Research* that his work had shown that feeding tea to mice 'markedly reduced' skin cancers. Further studies using rats and mice have indicated that the risks of contracting cancer from the carcinogens commonly found in cooked meat and fish can be reduced by drinking tea. Dr John Weisburger, director emeritus of the American Health Foundation, is so convinced of the cancer-halting properties of tea that he now recommends people to drink six cups a day. (It should be drunk black and relatively cool, as tests have shown that both milk and excessive heat seem to undermine the results.) It is good to see Western scientists in their large, expensively equipped laboratories proving something that the Chinese have known intuitively for so long.

The reason why all this is so new to the West is that for many centuries China kept itself isolated from the rest of the world. Small inroads were made by Jesuit missionaries from the late sixteenth century and there had been a brief report by the

Franciscans in the fourteenth century, but it was not until the 1850s that Westerners arrived in China in any numbers. The barriers went up again during the Cultural Revolution, and it has only been in the last thirty years that the West has had access to the vast storehouses of information that make up traditional Chinese medicine. The Chinese have had over five thousand years to accumulate all this information, whereas the West has had to take it all on board in a matter of three decades.

Another remedy commonly used by Chinese herbalists, garlic, is now being proclaimed as an ally in the fight against the West's second major killer, heart disease. Trials carried out at Oxford University's Department of Public Health and Primary Care by Dr Andrew Neil showed that dried garlic powder preparations reduced blood cholesterol by 8 per cent and that fresh garlic, garlic extract or garlic oil reduced it by 15 per cent. The Chinese have prescribed garlic since at least 1500 BC in the prevention of dysentery and typhoid. Now, research is beginning to show that it also has anti-spasmodic, antiseptic, diuretic and expectorant properties.

The list of proven successes goes on. Extract of the root of the plant *Pueraria lobata* (Ge Gen in Chinese) has long been used to treat alcoholism in China. Present-day researchers at the Harvard Medical School in Boston have discovered that the plant contains two chemicals which suppress the appetite for alcohol. This, they say, makes it a much safer treatment for alcoholics than existing drugs such as Antabuse, which interfere with the way the body metabolizes alcohol and can lead to a build-up of toxins.

Another success story concerns the painful condition of eczema. The dermatology department at London's Great Ormond Street Hospital are so impressed with the results of herbal treatments that they have developed tea bags of Chinese herbs and a skin cream based on a traditional herbal prescription.

But Western medicine also has its part to play. Encouraging

results have been achieved by combining Chinese and Western medicine in the treatment of certain difficult conditions such as haemolytic disease (breaking up of red blood corpuscles), which is found in newborn babies, and sclerodems — fibrous tissue in hardened skin. New drugs of high efficacy and low toxicity have been developed from medicinal herbs. For instance, an extract of *Artemisia apiacia* (Qing Hao in Chinese) has been used to treat pernicious and cerebral malaria. Although it has only recently been taken seriously in the West, its medical properties were mentioned in a medical textbook from the Da-guan period (*c.* AD 1092).

Traditional Chinese medicine, including herbal medicine, provides primary healthcare for between a quarter and half the world's population. It is already practised in half a dozen National Health Service clinics in the United Kingdom. As you will have realized, this evidence of growing interest is based not on any whim but on results. In the mid-1980s there were only a handful of Chinese herbalists in the UK — now there are over five hundred. They don't need to advertise, because word of mouth provides with them all the business they can cope with. In the United States over $400 billion is spent annually on traditional Chinese medicine. Even in Germany, a much smaller country, the market is estimated at some $1.5 billion.

A number of pharmaceutical companies in the West are researching Chinese herbal remedies for a range of diseases. Unfortunately most of them are looking at these remedies from a Western perspective, identifying the active ingredient and trying to tweak it in a molecular sense to obtain a new chemical entity. The problem is that they will end up with just another Western medicine, standardized to suit a whole range of patients. Chinese herbalists adjust every remedy to suit the patient's needs as they improve, or as they encounter new conditions of the illness. It is a time-consuming, labour-intensive way of practising medicine, which requires great patience and individual care. Perhaps this is why Chinese herbal medicine is so difficult to replicate chemically: to do so would deny the essential factor of the practitioner's input, which is an unpackageable ingredient.

However, conventional Western medicine and Chinese medicine should be seen as complementary to each other, rather than as alternatives. Herbalists are now beginning to get a lot more referrals from GPs. As a result they are being supplied with a detailed medical history of the client so that the two practitioners can work in conjunction. In the last few years the number of referrals has increased dramatically, as has the number of Western clients they see. In the UK three years ago herbalists saw very few Westerners, but now over 70 per cent of their clients are non-Chinese.

Both types of medicine have their advantages and drawbacks, which is why they need to work hand in hand for optimal results. Western medicine is usually more concrete in diagnosis and judgement. Treatment is often quicker, particularly in acute cases, and surgery is its strength. Its weak points are that it sees disease as something to be measured and quantified and often ignores the psychological, social and behavioural factors involved in illness.

Chinese medicine, on the other hand, can be too flexible and too general where diagnosis and judgement are concerned, and sometimes relies too heavily on the individual experiences of the practitioner. Its strong points are its highly flexible approach, enabling treatments to be changed as the patient improves, and its stress on preventative medicine. The Chinese way tends to treat the whole body rather than to try to isolate a particular infected area. And, finally, the herbs themselves, compared with chemically produced medicines, are relatively cheap and easy to use. They have minimal side-effects, and most have been tried and tested for over three thousand years.

Together, Chinese and Western medicine could form the most effective disease treatment the world has ever known.

1

The Principles of Traditional Chinese Medicine

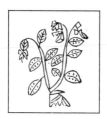

The way the Chinese see the human body, its make-up, its workings and its fundamental construction, is so different from Western medicine's view that one could almost be talking about two different species. To understand the principles of Chinese medicine you need a basic understanding of Daoism, the religion of China. The name comes from the Dao (pronounced: *dow*), which can be translated and understood, as 'The Way'. The Chinese say that everything is the Dao, everything is the Way. The Dao cannot really be likened to our Western concept of God, more to the idea of a fundamental inspiration from which everything in the universe flows. To Daoists everything can be divided into heaven and creation, or spirit and matter. Heaven is represented as a circle, and creation, sitting in the middle of heaven, as a square.

YIN AND YANG

From heaven, spirit, the circle was reduced to an unbroken line called yang, while creation, matter, became a broken line called yin.

Yin   Yang

The yin/yang symbolism was further developed into the best-known of all Chinese symbols:

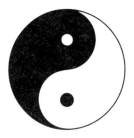

The yin/yang symbol

This is sometimes known as the Da Qi (T'ai Ch'i), the Supreme Ultimate or the Great Art. From the Supreme Ultimate comes the Dao, from the Dao comes yang and yin and from those two opposites there is everything in balance. Although the yang and yin are sometimes seen as opposites, each always contains an element of the other. This is why there is always the tiny dot of white within the black yin, and the tiny dot of dark within the white of the yang.

This division of everything into yin and yang is a very important concept — probably the most fundamental building-block upon which Chinese medicine is based. Within the human body the energy that maintains it and keeps it healthy can also be seen as incorporating the vital elements of yin and yang, as does the body itself. When there is an imbalance of yin and yang − too much of one or the other − illness can result, and herbal practitioners see their role as restoring that balance. By careful and detailed application of herbs and their chemical properties, which also contain that delicate balance, correct yin and yang can be restored within the human body. Each herb used is classified as either yin or yang.

It may be helpful to understand all the elements of yin and yang in order to appreciate how a herbalist sets about making a diagnosis.

	Yin	*Yang*
World	inner	outer
	down	up
	north	south
	matter	spirit
	creation	heaven
	earth	sky
	negative	positive
	passive	active
	female	male
	receptive	creative
	dark	light
	night	day
	cold	heat
	soft	hard
	wet	dry
	winter	summer
	shadow	sunshine
Body	interior	surface
	abdomen	back
	chest	spine

	Yin	*Yang*
	blood	qi energy (see page 18)
	cloudy body fluids	clear body fluids
Disease	chronic	acute
	non-active	virulent
	moist	dry
	retiring	advancing
	lingering	hasty
	weak	powerful
	decaying	flourishing
	patient feels cold	patient feels hot
	skin cold to touch	skin hot to touch
	low temperature	high temperature
	shivering	feverish

This list is by no means exhaustive, since everything in heaven and on earth is classified, by the Chinese, as either yin or yang. The problem that most Westerners have is that they tend to see yin and yang only as two extremes — something is either yin/female or yang/male. The Chinese, however, are always aware of the seed of the yang in the yin and the seed of the yin in the yang: nothing is ever only one or the other, and there is always a balance within the thing itself. A man might be described as yin, but that wouldn't make him a woman — merely someone who was in touch with his yin or female side. Likewise a woman might be described as yang; that wouldn't make her a man, but would just describe the type of woman she was — out-going, creative, active and dynamic.

The yin/yang symbol can also be used to represent the human body, with the head at the top representing spirit, yang, and the body below standing for matter, yin. Yang is the left-hand side of the body, while the right-hand side is female. It is interesting that more and more research is being done in the West into the two brain halves: the left brain controls the right side, would seem also to govern the more intuitive, artistic side of our nature, and is known as the female brain, while the right brain controls the left side, governs our more mathematical thought processes, and is known as the male brain. Western science is just discovering this; the Chinese apparently knew it five thousand years ago.

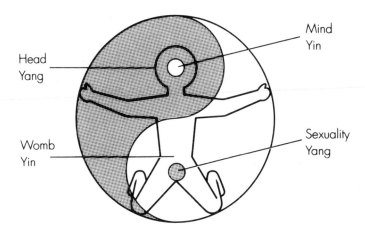

The yin/yang symbol with human body

Yin grows from yang, yang grows from yin, and neither can exist without the other. The abilities of the human body are seen as yang, while food, the energy source, is seen as yin. The body depends on the food to enable it to live, and yet to obtain the energy from the food it must be acted upon by the digestive system of the body.

The various organs and systems of the human body are constantly active, and so energy is constantly being needed and depleted. Too much need or too much depletion can both result in illness. For example, a weakening of yin and an over-expansion of yang could result in high blood pressure with the symptoms of dizziness, headache, short temper, sleeplessness, irritability, a tight pulse which is slower than normal and a red tongue. Obviously too much or too little food — yin — can result in excessive or insufficient yang.

The four seasons

Taking yin as winter, north, and yang as summer, south, we can combine these two symbols to create another two to represent east and west, respectively spring and autumn:

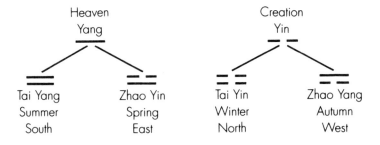

The two lines with seasons

The eight trigrams

From these four new symbols we can then produce another four to give us the rest of the compass and the mid-season points (you will notice that south is at the top, as is correct for a Chinese compass, and north at the bottom):

These are known as the eight trigrams (a trigram is three parallel lines).

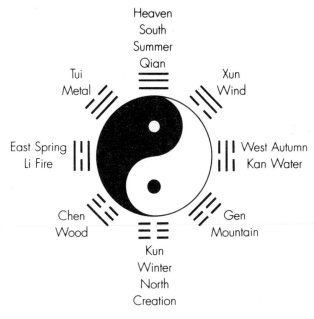

The eight trigrams (the Former Heaven Sequence)

- The top lines represent the duality of heaven and creation — the yin/yang
- The middle lines represent heaven and creation coming together to create the four seasons and the cardinal points of the compass
- The bottom lines represent us, people

The eight trigrams all have names, meanings, compass points and attributes:

Name		*Attributes/compass point*
Qian	– The Creative	heaven, south, summer
Tui	– The Lake	metal, south-east, joy
Li	– The Clinging	fire, east, spring, the sun

Name		Attributes/compass point
Chen	– The Arousing	wood, north-east, thunder
Kun	– The Receptive	creation, north, winter
Gen	– The Stillness	earth, north-west, mountain
Kan	– The Dangerous	water, west, autumn, the moon
Xun	– The Wind	gentle, south-west, wood

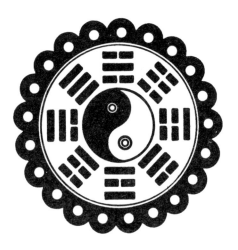

The Pah Kwa

The above symbol is known as the Pah Kwa, the Great Symbol, and is regarded as very lucky by the Chinese since it represents almost their entire spiritual and philosophical beliefs in one image.

The eight trigrams are thought to have been developed by Fu Xi, a legendary figure believed to have ruled around 3000 BC. It is said that he found the eight trigrams in the ornate markings on the shell of a tortoise which he studied on the banks of the Yellow River. The sequence in which he found them is called the Former Heaven Sequence, because around

1000 BC they were reputedly rearranged into what is known as the Later Heaven Sequence by King Wen, a philosopher and founder of the Zhou Dynasty.

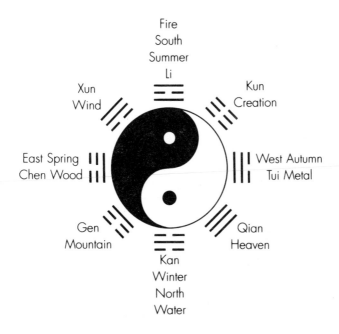

The Later Heaven Sequence

THE YI JING

These eight trigrams can be paired into sixty-four new symbols (eight multiplied by eight) called hexagrams, which use six lines. These sixty-four hexagrams each have a meaning; Fu Xi first wrote them down in a herbal and agricultural almanac which he called the *Yi Jing* (often spelt *I Ching* in the West and pronounced *ee ching*), or the *Book of Changes*. The only major restructuring was done by King Wen, who added to Fu Xi's interpretations.

THE FIVE ELEMENTS

The four cardinal points of the Later Heaven Sequence are also four elements:

- south/fire/li
- north/water/kan
- east/wood/chen
- west/metal/tui

The fifth element occupies the centre and is . . .

- earth

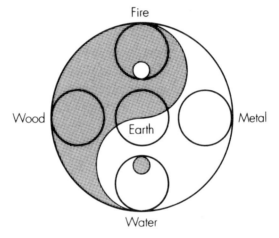

The five elements with earth in the centre

Most Oriental wisdom, medicine and philosophy is based on the Theory of the Five Aspects (*Wu Xing*) which suggests that, whilst we are a combination of all the elements or aspects, we each tend to display the characteristics of one more than the others. (These elements are not the elements of conventional Western astrology, and it is better to regard them more as aspects of character.)

Earth *Tu* The Diplomat

Moderate, sense of loyalty, harmonious, likes to belong, pays attention to details, likes company, needs to be needed, can be stubborn, should avoid damp.

Fire *Huo* The Magician

Compassionate, intuitive, communicative, likes pleasure, seeks excitement, likes to be in love, doesn't like to be bored, should avoid heat.

Water *Shui* The Philosopher

Imaginative, honest, clever, seeks knowledge, original, tough, independent, can be secretive, needs to be protected, should avoid cold.

Metal *Chin* The Catalyst

Organized, likes to control, precise, discriminating, needs to be right, likes order and cleanliness, appreciates quality, should avoid dryness.

Wood *Mu* The Pioneer

Expansive, purposeful, active, likes to be busy, can be domineering, needs to win, practical, should avoid wind.

Before making a diagnosis and formulating a prescription, it is essential that the herbalist knows which element most closely represents you.

Each of the different elements has contrasting responses to the others:

Earth	helps metal
	is helped by fire
	hinders water
	is hindered by wood
Fire	helps earth
	is helped by wood
	hinders metal
	is hindered by water
Water	helps wood

	is helped by metal
	hinders fire
	is hindered by earth
Metal	helps water
	is helped by earth
	hinders wood
	is hindered by fire
Wood	helps fire
	is helped by water
	hinders earth
	is hindered by metal

Each of these five elements rules or influences different internal organs, parts of the body, emotional expressions, colours, tastes and energies (see table opposite).

Each of the five elements is also indicative of very different type of person; for example earth types are large and well rounded with soft skin. They love good food. Being in charge is important to them but they are prone to worrying and can be interfering and over-protective. They can suffer from water retention, indigestion and muscular tenderness. Earth types are attentive, have good memories, and are supportive, caring and sympathetic.

Fire types have graceful hands and feet, with long necks, arms and hands. They often suffer from disturbed sleep, disorders of blood pressure and circulation, fainting and dizzy spells, and they can tire easily. Fire types love sensation and excitement and can be prone to drug abuse. They are tender, aware and sensitive.

Water types have strong lean bodies; they are prone to back problems, low sexual drive and can suffer from head-aches and lack of energy. They are articulate and clever with a thirst for knowledge. They can be emotionally reserved but are probably the most creative and imaginative of all the elements.

Element	Earth	Fire	Water	Metal	Wood
Zang internal organs	Spleen	Heart	Kidneys	Lungs	Liver
Fu internal organs	Stomach	Small intestine	Bladder	Large intestine	Gall Bladder
*Facial features**	Mouth	Tongue	Ears	Nose	Eyes
*Body**	Muscle	Pulse	Bones	Skin/hair	Tendons
Expression	Thought	Gaiety	Fright	Worry	Anger
Colour	Yellow	Red	Black	White	Green
Taste	Sweet	Bitter	Salt	Pungent	Sour
Energy	Wet	Hot	Cold	Pungent	Dry
Season	Late summer	Summer	Winter	Autumn	Spring
*Smell***	Fragrant	Scorched	Rotten	Putrid	Rancid
Direction	Centre	South	North	West	East

* These are the parts most prone to ailments

** The names for the smells may have lost a little in their translation.

13

Metal types tend to be small and delicate with fine features; they like order and reason; they have high standards; they can suffer from stiff joints, dry skin and hair and poor circulation; they can be very formal and reserved.

Wood people tend to be supple, muscular, strong and slim. They may suffer from high blood pressure. They may have vertigo and can be short-tempered, prone to sprained ankles and wrists, tension in the neck and across the shoulders, migraines and tension headaches, constipation and so on. They tend to be quick, decisive people, restless and impatient. They are usually competitive and impulsive. And their complaints can be easily and quickly recognized by a Chinese herbalist and treated accordingly.

These five elemental types are known as the Five Phase Theory and can be further categorized into the Harmony of the Five Sentiments — anger, joy, fear, sorrow and pensiveness — giving a total of twenty-five combinations. To keep the body healthy it is necessary to keep all these sentiments in balance.

THE HARMONY OF THE FIVE SENTIMENTS

Anger

If the emotion of anger dominates, the patient will be easily upset by frustrations, prone to violent outbursts, volatile and unpredictable. These people can be seen by others as self-controlled and self-disciplined, but when stress and tension build up they can explode into rage. Illnesses that they are prone to include ulcers, migraines and haemorrhoids. They also tend to suffer from 'hot' (yang, increased activity often revealing as fever) illnesses.

Sandra

At the age of forty-seven Sandra had been going through the menopause for the previous two years, suffering hot flushes and an extremely short temper. However her periods were still normal, as was her bowel function. Her tongue had red spots and a white fur known as 'white wall'.

On her first visit in June 1993 she was given a Chinese herbal patent medicine for menopause, consisting of five pills to be taken three times a day before meals for seven days. The ingredients were:

Bo He *Mentha arvensis (mint)*
Gan Jiang *Zingiber officinale* (ginger root)
Gan Cao *Glycyrrhiza uralensis* (liquorice root)
Dang Gui *Angelica sinensis* (Chinese angelica)
Bai Zhu *Atractylodes macrocephala*
Bai Shao *Paeoniae laciflora* (white peony root)
Chai Hu *Bupleurum chinense* (thorowax root)

This prescription was prepared with honey.

On her second visit, a fortnight later, she was much improved. She was sleeping better and the hot flushes had decreased. Her pulse was 'stable'. Her tongue was also better, with only the tip showing slight red spots, although the 'white wall' was still visible. Her temper had abated considerably, and she felt calmer and less likely to fly into a rage.

At the time of her third visit, after another two weeks, even more improvement was evident. No hot flushes had been experienced for seven days, and she was sleeping normally. The 'white wall' on her tongue had cleared up and it was pale, although showing visible teeth marks (indicating a soft flaccid tongue with no firmness). Her pulse was still stable.

Sandra was prescribed the same herbal medicine twice daily for three weeks, at the end of which time all her symptoms had cleared up and she was considered discharged.

Joy

When joy is the main motivating force in a person's life they are liable to suffer extreme mood swings: they're either up or down, never in between. They can become endless pleasure-seekers. They crave excitement, and feel empty and alone without it. Typical illnesses can include anorexia, schizophrenia, manic-depressive psychosis and hypoglycaemia.

Fear

People who live their lives in fear can become isolated, hermit-like and withdrawn, cutting themselves off from the world in their belief that it is a fundamentally evil place which wants to harm them. They imagine the worst-case scenario in everything they do. Illnesses can include deafness, arthritis and senility.

Sorrow

This kind of person will avoid excitement or any emotional involvement so as to protect themselves from the emotion they fear most: sorrow. They believe that is what they deserve, and subsequently shut themselves off from the world of relationships. They like to control everyone around them, so that no one can hurt them. Illnesses manifest as constipation, frigidity and asthma.

Pensiveness

These patients get bogged down in minutiae and worry over little details to the point of obsession. They like security and safety and can become lethargic and apathetic when faced with new challenges, mainly because it is all too much for them. Illnesses tend to show up as obesity, poor digestion, heart problems and high blood pressure.

THE IMPORTANCE OF HOT AND COLD

For a Western doctor it may be sufficient to know that a patient has flu, but a Chinese doctor will want to know if your flu is hot or cold, wet or dry. Even sweating will be classified as either hot or cold. This information is vital if the right herbs or combination of herbs are to be prescribed.

If we suffer from a hot fever, our herbalist will prescribe a cooling herb to counteract the heat. Similarly, if we have a shivering cold we will be treated with a heating herb to warm us. Examples are Da Zheng Qi Soup (made with rhubarb, sodium sulphate and magnolia), which reduces high temperatures, thirst, headaches, delirium and vomiting; and Warm Spleen Soup (Chinese angelica, dried ginger and liquorice) which is used to treat coldness, especially in the limbs and spleen, and constipation caused by cold. (See Pernicious Influences.)

ENERGY, BLOOD, MERIDIANS AND INTERNAL ORGANS

When prescribing medicines Chinese herbalists take four major factors into consideration:

- qi (energy)
- blood and other body fluids

17

- meridians (channels)
- internal organs

QI

Chinese philosophy allocates yin or yang qualities to everything and believes in an energy that binds them all together and flows within and around them. The Chinese call it qi (pronounced *chee* and sometimes spelt ch'i) and regard it as one of the four most important aspects of Chinese herbal medicine. When qi flows well there is harmony and balance, but when it stagnates it is the cause of many illnesses. It can be seen as the principle that underlies the Dao – the invisible force that animates everything, the life force. We cannot see, touch, taste, hear or feel qi, but we are aware of its effect. Creation is qi taking shape. When we die, the living qi leaves our bodies. qi is the original breath which gives life to the inanimate body. It is expended throughout life, and the essence of traditional Chinese medicine is to keep the qi as complete as possible. It is through strengthening qi that healing takes place.

The way qi flows in and around our dwellings is called feng shui. Feng shui can be seen as a way of aligning both our dwellings and ourselves to receive the maximum benefit of good qi. Feng shui means, literally, *wind* and *water*. It is an extremely ancient and well developed system dating back in China at least three thousand years but it has only become known in the West in the last century.

If you lived in China and wanted to move house you would call in your feng shui consultant (*feng shui xian-sheng*). They would come and see the new house, take measurements using a feng shui compass called a *Lo-pan*. Also they would need your birth date, place and time so they could draw up a detailed eight-point horoscope to see if you and your proposed new dwelling were compatible. And finally they would need a detailed report of all the previous occupants of the house with a history of how their luck, wealth, health and happiness fared while they were living there.

When they had all the information necessary they would compile a report on the feng shui of your proposed new house. This report would include such details as:

- the *lung mei* (dragon's veins) of qi energy flowing in and around the building
- whether your family would prosper or decline there
- what changes you would need to make to increase your wealth there or to counteract any bad luck
- whether it was a yin or yang dwelling

On the basis of their report you would decide whether to move there or not. The Chinese consider it easier to put right construction faults than to buy a house that has a long established bad feng shui because of its poor siting.

So what if the report is unfavourable? Well, there are a lot of fairly simple remedies that can be carried out such as:

- hanging strategic mirrors to deflect sha (unhealthy energy)
- changing the layout of the garden
- adding or moving plants inside the house
- changing colour schemes
- using bamboo flutes, ribbons, statues and even electrical equipment to alter the flow of qi
- using wind chimes, flags and fountains to break up stagnant qi.

All these can help the flow of qi. There are four types of qi:

- **Sheng qi** – growing qi from the east
- **Yang qi** – nourishing qi from the south
- **Zang qi** – hidden qi from the north
- **Sha qi** – disruptive qi from the west

Now you can see the connection between the compass directions, yin and yang, and qi. When the qi is disruptive (*sha*) it can cause ill health. Herbs can help correct the imbalance, but it may sometimes be necessary to move house completely. At your initial consultation the herbalist will ask many questions, including where and how you live. This information is useful in making a diagnosis, as the Chinese know well that nothing works in isolation: we are all connected with everyone and everything else. In Chinese medicine qi is regarded as a yang force, the source of growth and disintegration, the prime mover and consolidating force of the blood. It organizes the whole body, repels attack from outside and promotes the functioning of the internal organs.

Within the body qi is further categorized into four types:

Original qi

Sometimes known as real or correct qi, it represents the strengths and weaknesses of the body in combating all forms of illness. If the original qi is weak, infection can take hold; restoring original qi will ward off illness.

Internal organ qi

This is the specific energy of particular organs: there is qi of the liver, qi of the heart, qi of the lungs, and so on. The combined qi of the stomach and spleen is known as central qi. If this becomes weakened it causes difficulties in the function of the digestive system, a slowing down in the rate of mental activity, weak voice and problems with the uterus. These conditions must be treated by a method which strengthens central qi. The qi of the lungs and heart together is known as ancestral qi and assists respiration and circulation. If the ancestral qi is weakened, it causes a weak heartbeat and problems with breathing.

Guarding qi

This surrounds all the meridians or channels (see page 24) and is dispersed throughout the whole body. It travels outside the meridians and is regarded as the boundary fence of all internal systems.

Protein qi

This type of qi travels within the pulse meridians and provides vital protein to the blood. Guarding qi and protein qi work very closely together, one outer and the other inner.

The disruption of qi

Qi can be disrupted in three ways: weakening, stagnating and mischannelling.

Weakening qi

This means that there is insufficient energy, and is most noticeable when the qi of the lungs and the spleen are weakened. The symptoms are loss of appetite, reluctance to speak, sweating for no apparent reason, dizzy spells and a feeble pulse.

Stagnation of qi

This occurs when the mechanism of internal organ functioning meets an obstruction to its normal operation, and is found mainly in the spleen, lungs and liver. Stagnation of qi in the lungs results in tightness of the chest, pain, wheezy breathing and too much phlegm. Symptoms can include tightness in the chest, sides and abdomen, accompanied by pain.

Qi stagnating in the liver produces a bloated abdomen, abdominal pain, and in women a painful menstrual cycle with irregular periods. Stagnant spleen qi produces indigestion and a painful, swollen abdomen. Stagnation of qi in the meridian veins will result in aching in the muscles and joints of all limbs, sometimes with swelling.

Mischannelling of qi

Each organ's qi flows in a particular direction, and if that direction gets reversed illness can result. The stomach and lung qi flow downwards, for instance: upward flowing lung qi would cause asthma and coughs, and upward-flowing stomach qi would produce vomiting and nausea. Reversed liver qi would cause vomiting of blood, fainting and unconsciousness.

BLOOD

Whereas qi is seen as yang, blood is seen as yin: the two provide a nourishing balance and complement each other. They are both equally necessary for a healthy body. 'Blood gives birth to qi, but qi rules the blood' runs an old Chinese saying. The motivating energy of qi encourages the blood to flow. If the qi stagnates, the blood clots. If there is an inadequate supply of blood, loss of sensitivity and even paralysis can result.

Illnesses related to the blood can be divided into three main categories: escape, weakness and clotting.

Escape of the blood

Blood escaping from any of the major organs can be caused by a number of factors which would have to be examined independently. The vomiting of blood, for example, would be seen very differently from excessive menstrual bleeding. Normal bleeding from cuts and wounds would be seen not as escape of the blood, but as injuries.

Weakness of the blood

Symptoms of weak blood can include: pallor of the lips, yellowish skin colour, pale tongue and nails, blurred sight, dizziness, fainting spells and exhaustion. Anaemia is an example. Restoring qi can strengthen the blood.

If there has been a heavy loss of blood, then the body's natural ability to manufacture blood may be impaired. Blood transfusions are a new idea in China, as the Chinese have always regarded blood as precious and not to be given away.

Clotting of blood

Qi stagnating can cause the blood to clot; if this occurs in the lungs, then the patient may well cough up blood. Blood clotting is most commonly seen in the form of bruising, which is usually treated by massage, often with cold water. Ice can be used to good effect. Blood clotting may be caused by internal bleeding and can develop in the veins of the heart. It can also occur in the limbs or lungs and can be very painful, affecting movement. Blood clotting, as in thrombosis, can be extremely serious.

Spirit (sperm)

In Chinese medicine 'spirit' has two meanings. It is a term for the vital force of the cells which is required for human growth, but it also means sperm. Spirit is normally seen as being stored in the kidneys, and a part of this, the Chinese believe, becomes sperm.

Juices and dew

Body fluid is divided into two categories: the fluid that is dispersed between the joints and in the brain is known as *juices*, whereas the fluid dispersed among the internal organs, skin and muscles is called *dew*. All body fluids, even tears and sweat, are known as either juices or dew. Blood and dew are seen as closely related, even as coming from one source, and patients with a blood loss condition would never be treated with a sudorific (medicine to promote sweating).

Phlegm is a form of dew which the Chinese say is developed in the spleen and stored in the lungs. When excessive phlegm is produced in the lungs in such conditions as asthma it cannot settle properly. A remedy would be prescribed that would either disperse or expel the phlegm.

THE MERIDIANS

The body contains a balance of yin and yang and the flow of qi. Qi is said to flow along lines known as meridians. Most Chinese medicine works by accepting that the meridians conduct energy; these lines are used by acupuncturists and are illustrated in acupuncture charts.

In acupuncture treatment, needles are inserted at several points along a single meridian. An additional needle may be inserted at the point of greatest pain, specific to the indvidual, which may or may not be along the same meridian. This point of greatest pain is known as the Hua Tuo after a famous doctor of that name.

The main difference between acupuncture and herbal medicine is that acupuncture is concerned with stimulating and improving the flow of energy along the meridians, whereas herbal medicine is more concerned with balancing the yin and yang of the major body organs. Even so, acupuncture and herbal medicine are frequently used alongside each other (see page 47).

The Twelve Meridians

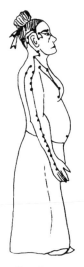

Sanjiao

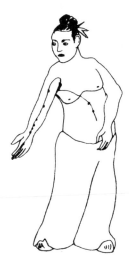

Pericardium

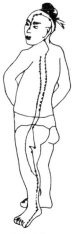

Bladder

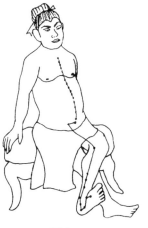

Kidney

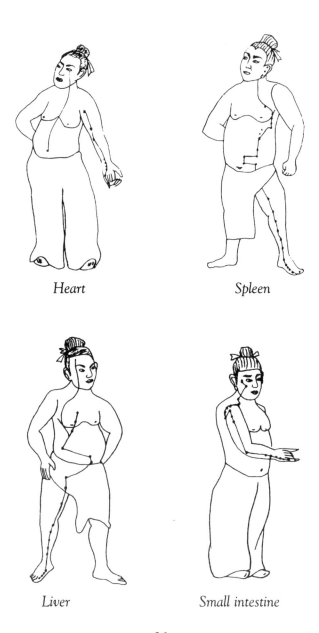

Heart

Spleen

Liver

Small intestine

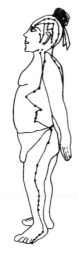

Gall bladder

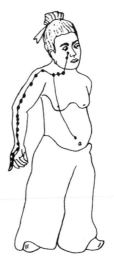

Large intestine

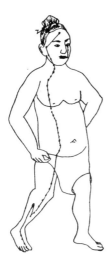

Stomach

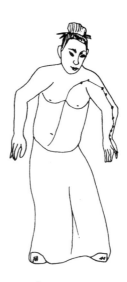

Lung

The Jin Mai

The twelve real meridians form a complete circulatory system around the body: hand/lung (great yin) → hand/large intestine (yang) → foot/stomach (yang) → foot/spleen (yin) → hand/heart (yin) → hand/small intestine (yang) → foot/bladder (yang) → foot/kidney (yin) → hand/pericardium (yin) → hand/Sanjiao (yang) → foot/gall bladder (yang) → foot/liver (yin) → hand/lung (great yin).

Each of the meridians has collateral or accompanying channels located in other parts of the body; for example, the hand/large intestine (yang) channel has collateral channels in the lungs. These collateral channels could be seen as the branches of a tree and the meridian as the trunk.

Each meridian and its collaterals are linked with particular illnesses and their treatment.

The three yin hand channels

Channel	Collateral channels	Illnesses
Hand/lung (great yin)	Large intestine	Lung, throat and chest complaints
Hand/heart (yin)	Small intestine	Heart, stomach and chest complaints, diarrhoea, mental disorders, asthma
Hand/pericardium (yin)	Sanjiao	Chest diseases, mental disorder, apoplexy

The Circular Meridian System

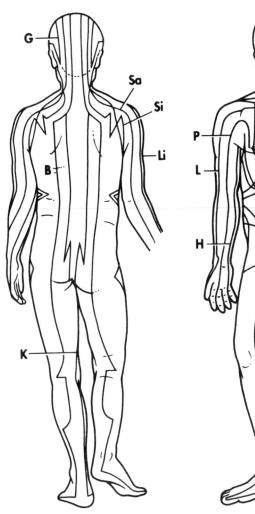
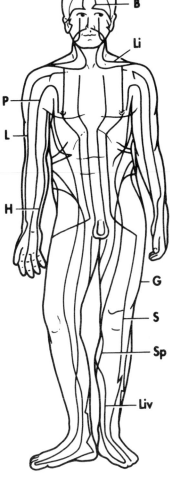

L	= Lung	**P**	= Pericardium
Li	= Large Intestine	**B**	= Bladder
S	= Stomach	**K**	= Kidney
Sp	= Spleen	**Sa**	= Sanjiao
H	= Heart	**G**	= Gall Bladder
Si	= Small Intestine	**Liv**	= Liver

The three yang hand channels

Channel	Collateral channels	Illnesses
Hand/large intestine (yang)	Lungs	High fever, high blood pressure, ear, nose and throat problems, complaints of the chest and abdomen, tooth decay
Hand/Sanjiao (yang)	Wall of the heart	Constipation and complaints of the ear, nose and throat
Hand/small intestine (yang)	Heart	Mental disorders, high fever, complaints of the neck and shoulders, eye disorders

The three yang foot channels

Channel	Collateral channels	Illnesses
Foot/stomach (yang)	Spleen	Face, mouth, teeth, throat
Foot/gall bladder (yang)	Liver	Liver, gall bladder, eyes, ears, throat
Foot/bladder (yang)	Kidneys	Back of the neck, back, top of the skull, eyes

The three yin foot channels

Channel	Collateral channels	Illnesses
Foot/spleen (yin)	Stomach	Stomach disorders, loss of sleep, bleeding
Foot/liver (yin)	Gall bladder	Liver, gall-bladder
Foot/kidney (yin)	Bladder	Mental disorders, depression

The meridian channels

One of the main differences between Western and Chinese medicine is the interpretations of the *meridians*. These, according to Chinese medicine, are the channels along or through which the qi energy flows. Western medicine is only recently beginning to recognise the meridians whereas the Chinese have studied, understood and used them for as long as they have practised medicine.

There are twelve pairs of channels, they are found on both sides of the body and correspond on left and right sides. There are three yin hand channels, three yin foot channels, three yang hand channels and three yang foot channels. These are called the twelve Jin Mai or meridians. These twelve each relate to a specific internal organ. The Chinese include the Sanjiao, the triple-warmer which is the three portions of the body cavity, in their classification as an internal organ.

The Sanjiao

The three body cavities are collectively called the Sanjiao in classical Chinese medicine and can be seen as the upper, middle and lower. The upper is the area around the heart and lungs and corresponds roughly to the chest. The middle is the area around the spleen and stomach and the lower is the area around the kidneys, liver, intestine and bladder. Their respective functions are: upper – receiving; middle – transporting; lower – passing or eliminating.

INTERNAL ORGANS

The Zang Fu

The internal organs of Chinese medicine are collectively called the Zang Fu and are not to be confused with Western medicine's similar-sounding organs. The Chinese see the Zang Fu as a complete, interdependent system of organs, meridians and qi flowing through and between them. Even their function is seen differently.

The internal organs are divided into twelve:

- six Fu: large intestine, small intestine, stomach, bladder, gall bladder and Sanjiao (the triple warmer or three body cavities)
- Special Permanent Fu: brain, marrow, bones, veins, and womb
- six Zang: kidneys, spleen, heart, lungs, liver and pericardium (known as the heart-protector)

The twelve Zang Fu and the Special Permanent Fu form a complete system and are all seen as working together to create a healthy body, although each constituent has its separate function. The two groups, Zang and Fu, are responsible for the two main tasks of the human body: preserving and storing energy (qi), and digestion and elimination of waste.

The six Zang collectively have the task of energy collection, storage and distribution. The six Fu are, in general, responsible for sorting out useful from useless substances and for getting rid of waste. Again, don't confuse their functions, descriptions or names with those of conventional Western medicine. Whereas there may well be similarities and overlaps, the differences are probably greater.

Functions and abilities of the six Zang

Combined function	Preserves energy (qi)
Heart	Rules pulse and spirit
Liver	Rules tendons and passages. Reservoir of blood
Spleen	Rules the circulatory systems, including blood, skin and muscles
Lungs	Rules qi, energy and air. Forces clearance of passages. Preserves the skin and hair
Kidneys	Preserves spirit (sperm). Rules bone and water. Provides bone marrow (includes the brain)
Pericardium	Protects the heart. Governs sex

Functions and abilities of the six Fu

Combined function	Reception, digestion, distribution and elimination of waste
Stomach	Receives food and liquids
Small intestine	Digests and receives food. Separates different forms of energy usage
Large intestine	Passes wastes
Bladder	Acts as reservoir and passer of urine
Sanjiao	Transports food and liquids. Passes wastes
Gall bladder	Preserves and stores gall juice

Functions and abilities of the Special Permanent Fu

Combined function	Conservation of qi
Brain	Mental control. Commands all functions
Marrow	Manufactures bones
Veins (pulses)	Circulates blood
Womb	Commands female reproductive and menstrual system

The yin and yang of the Zang Fu

Each of the six Zang internal organs is regarded as yin, and the six Fu organs as yang. The Zang are the solid organs which store, while the Fu are the hollow organs which transform. As there is always a balance of yin and yang, each member of the Zang and Fu is linked with a corresponding organ in the other:

Yin (Zang)	Yang (Fu)
Heart	Small intestine
Liver	Gall bladder
Spleen	Stomach
Lung	Large intestine
Kidneys	Bladder
Pericardium	Sanjiao

The five elements of the Zang Fu

Each of these internal organs is also governed by, or comes under the influence of, one of the five elements:

Ruling element	Yin organ	Yang organ
Wood	Liver	Gall bladder
Fire	Heart	Small intestine
Earth	Spleen	Stomach
Metal	Lungs	Large intestine
Water	Kidneys	Bladder
Fire	Pericardium	Sanjiao

And each of the elements correspond to one of the members of the Harmony of the Five Sentiments (see page 14):

Wood	Anger	Liver gall bladder
Fire	Joy	Pericardium/Sanjiao/heart/ small intestine
Earth	Pensiveness	Spleen/stomach
Water	Fear	Kidneys/bladder
Metal	Sorrow	Lungs/large intestine

For Westerners these ideas may seem strange at first, but they do have parallels in Western beliefs. For example, when someone is angry we say they are full of bile or bitterness; when someone is full of joy or love then they have a 'full heart'; when someone is worried or pensive they may well feel it in the pit of their stomach; when someone is frightened their bladder often needs frequent emptying; and when someone is sad or sorrowful you can hear it in their lungs as they sigh deeply. Herbal practitioners know all this and much more besides, and use it to determine which element you may be and which sentiment you predominantly exhibit. In this way they can determine the cause of your complaint and which herb combination to treat you with or which meridian may need adjustment.

Liu Yin

The six Pernicious Influences, also known as the Six Evils, are not in fact evil — just natural events that only become harmful when the body cannot adjust quickly enough or strongly enough to them. They are:

- dryness
- dampness
- heat (or fire)
- cold
- wind
- summer heat

When the balance of yin and yang are upset, then the harmful effects of the Pernicious Influences can be manifested. Qi protects the body from Liu Yin but when, for whatever reason, qi becomes weakened, illness can develop. Fever, body aches, chills and general discomfort are the signs that Liu Yin is gaining hold.

When there is actual climatic Liu Yin, such as weather conditions, it is known as External Pernicious Influence; but there is also Internal Pernicious Influence, where the internal organs become weakened or malfunction. Internal Pernicious Influence illnesses are usually chronic, whereas External Pernicious Influence illnesses are acute and much more sudden. Fever or chills seldom accompany Internal Pernicious Influence illnesses.

Dryness (zao)

Dryness Pernicious Influence is usually associated with autumn and is a yang influence. Dryness is linked to dehydration, and its symptoms are dry lips, nostrils and tongue, cracked skin and dry bowel motions.

External Dryness Pernicious Influence can be revealed by a dry cough with little phlegm, asthma and chest pain or a tightness of the chest, as it often interferes with the descending and circulating functions of the lungs.

Dampness (shi)

Dampness is associated with the 'long summer' which is a yin influence as it is heavy, slow and wet. It is associated with any damp weather or damp conditions. Its symptoms are loss of appetite, indigestion, nausea, diarrhoea with heavy, sticky bowel motions, cloudy urine, a feeling of heaviness, a 'thick' head, heavy and sore limbs and oozing skin eruptions.

External Dampness will come on suddenly, whereas Internal Dampness is much slower; but they are both lingering, stagnating influences which are difficult to shift and can last a long time. The spleen is most sensitive to dampness, which is why most of the symptoms affect the digestive process.

Mucus (tan) is seen as a form of internal dampness; mucus is regarded differently by the Chinese from the way it is viewed in Western medicine – it is seen as not just a fluid in the lungs but also as mucus of the heart, which can cause mental instability, and mucus of the meridians, which can cause numbness or even paralysis.

Heat (re) or fire (huo)

Heat is seen as the External Pernicious Influence here and Fire as the Internal one. Heat is associated with summer and is a yang influence. Its symptoms are high fever, skin inflammation, boils, carbuncles, a cough with thick yellow phlegm, dry tongue, unusual thirst, dry bowel motions or burning sensations in the anus, only small quantities of urine, delirium, headache with swollen throat and soreness.

Cold (han)

Cold is associated with winter and is a yin influence. It affects the meridians and can block the flow of qi and blood. Its symptoms are sharp, cramp-like pains that respond to the application of heat, shivering, a bluish tinge to the skin, slow movements, pronounced chills and chronic under-activity. Coldness manifests through the kidneys, and the fluids affected by cold conditions − such as mucus, urine, sweat, vomit and diarrhoea − are seen as watery, cool, transparent or clear.

Wind (feng)

Wind is a yang influence; both within and outside the body it is regarded in the same way. It is associated with spring and with movement, change and urgency. Its symptoms are pains that move from place to place, skin eruptions that appear and reappear in different locations, spasms and tremors, dizziness and twitching, sudden headaches, sore and itchy throat, congested nasal passages, numbness of the limbs, and even convulsions and seizures. Wind Pernicious Influence manifesting as an internal influence affects the liver.

Summer heat (shu)

Summer Heat Pernicious Influence is always an external influence. It is brought on by exposure to extreme heat, which damages qi and causes exhaustion, sudden high fever, heavy sweating and loss of fluids. It is often associated with Dampness Pernicious Influence.

As you will now be aware, the holistic view of Chinese practitioners is that everything is linked − everything is interdependent on everything else within the human body. Even the outside of the body is regarded as yang, while the inside is yin. Life and death are seen as yang, while birth and growth are yin. The Chinese herbal practitioner always strives to restore the balance, the harmony, between yin and yang, and knows that each change will subtly alter other parts of the human body.

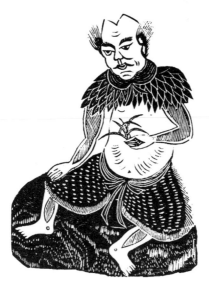

The Chinese Medicine God

2

The Role of Herbalism Within the Chinese Tradition

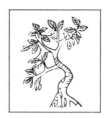

THE HISTORY OF CHINESE HERBAL MEDICINE

For as long as humans have existed, certain members of every community have noticed that some berries, roots, flowers, stems or leaves produce particular effects. Someone eats a berry and it makes them vomit; someone who is constipated eats a certain flower stem and finds that they suddenly have normal bowel function; someone else eats a root and quickly shakes off a lethargy that had been there for weeks. It all gets noticed, recorded (either orally or written down) and added to the stock of tribal or communal folklore.

The so-called Chinese Yellow Emperor, Huang Ti, is supposed to have discovered the secrets of herbal medicine, and then to have invented writing so as to record his findings.

He reigned, it is said, from 2696 to 2598 BC, and is also credited with having invented wheeled vehicles, armour, ships and pottery. He is generally regarded as the third of China's first five rulers, known as the Five August Ones. His story is part legend, part fact, but his book the *Huang-ti Nei Qing Su Wen* (The Yellow Emperor's Classic of Internal Medicine) most certainly does exist. Although most of it was not written down fully until around 200–100 BC parts of it appear to date back to the Shang dynasty (c. 1523–1028 BC), and there is some evidence that Huang Ti is based on a real person – a powerful religious and political leader who imposed certain codes of law and possibly also of religion on his people – who lived in the Yellow River basin in China.

The book consists of a dialogue between Huang Ti and one of his ministers, Qi Po, in which the Emperor asks questions and the minister gives answers in the form of long discourses which cover not only medicine but also diet, lifestyle, moral codes, hygiene and ethics. More than just a textbook, it is a manual for living, including social and religious instruction. It covers such topics as the Dao, yin and yang, the five elements and the system of numbers, the celestial stems, anatomical and physiological concepts, diagnosis, diseases, therapeutic concepts, acupuncture and moxibustion. Still in print, and still in everyday use in both China and the West, it is one of the oldest medical textbooks in existence.

Others followed. For example, in 1973 a 2100-year-old tomb in China's Hunan Province was opened and found to contain a set of medical textbooks printed on silk. They outlined the principles of Chinese medicine, including pulse-taking, yin and yang and diagnostic techniques.

The regulating of Chinese medicine is first recorded about the time that the *Huang-ti Nei Qing Su Wen* was being compiled. In the *Qian Han Shu* (AD 100) and the *Hou Han Shou* (AD 450) – the Books of the Han, which are the dynastic records of the Han period (207 BC–AD 220) – medical books were separated into four classifications:

- *Yi Jing*: concerned with the internal structures of the body and the causes of illness (not to be confused with the *Yi Jing* or *Book of Changes*. 'Yi' means 'medical')
- *Qing Fang*: herbal prescriptions and remedies
- *Fang Zhong*: sexual techniques and health
- *Shen Qian*: ways of gaining immortality

Some thirty-six books are recorded in these categories. The number of classifications had increased to thirteen by the time of the Ming dynasty (1368–1644), but by the Qing (1644–1912) it had been reduced to nine which were recognized by the Imperial Medical College. During the sixteenth century Li Shizhen, a famous and respected naturalist, compiled a 52-volume encyclopaedia which described nearly two thousand medicines and eleven thousand prescriptions, and covered such topics as geology, botany, chemistry and zoology.

Herbal medicine has always had an important place in China's medical history, with the exception of the early years of the Republic from 1912, when it entered its only period of decline. Then it was ridiculed and scorned by the intellectuals, who were only interested in conventional Western medicine. In some cases it was an offence to practise herbal medicine. It declined right up to the time of the Communist Revolution, when it was again needed. Since 1949 the Chinese have worked hard to keep the best of traditional herbal medicine as well as making use of the best of Western medicine. Today in China rural doctors receive training in both disciplines, and doctors practising Western medicine are encouraged to study traditional Chinese medicine. In 1955 the China Academy of Traditional Chinese Medicine was set up as one of three major research institutes affiliated to the Ministry of Public Health. Nearly two hundred smaller institutes are also researching and evaluating the role of Chinese medicine in diagnosis, treatment and the understanding of disease processes, with promising results. When Western medicine has finished evaluating and researching traditional Chinese medicine to its own satisfaction, it will be ready to put both into place alongside each other.

TRAINING REQUIRED

Throughout the ages Daoism and herbal medicine have gone hand in hand in China. It has been estimated that, for every official doctor trained in herbal medicine and working from the great textbooks, there were at least ten Taoist priests practising the art. As often as not these people were illiterate and working entirely from handed down knowledge.

In China today there are several different types of herbalist: those who have no formal medical training, those who are formally trained and those who are a mixture of both. Many of those without any training are called barefoot doctors, and they tend to practise in the more remote rural areas. Those with a formal training leading to a qualification such as a degree, tend to operate more in the cities.

In the West the legal requirements vary from country to country, and even, where applicable, from state to state. In several European countries no one can practise any form of medicine without a conventional medical training, although there are many unlicensed herbalists who, whilst operating essentially outside the law, are nevertheless dispensing openly. In the USA the situation varies from state to state: a few allow herbalists to practise with no formal training, but most require a medical qualification. In the UK there is no legal requirement for qualification, although that situation may change in the near future. For specific details of training and herbal suppliers see Useful Addresses.

Before seeking treatment it is best to satisfy yourself as to the legal requirements of the country you live in, the qualifications you expect and the type of premises and practice you will feel happy with. Most large cities have a Chinatown where you will find Chinese herbalists. A personal recommendation is always preferable, but in the absence of this you can always carry out a personal survey. Go to each one and see how it feels. Is it clean and wholesome? Are the herbs healthy-looking? Does the herbalist seem friendly and helpful? Do they make you feel confident? Is the business only recently started, or has the practitioner been there for a number of years?

THE USE OF HERBS

Herbs play a large part in the Chinese diet: they are used in cooking in much the same way as people in the West use salt or pepper. But the Chinese have a much larger repertoire of herbs to use and know which ones to add or leave out of their cooking according to the circumstances. An older branch of Chinese herbal medicine was known literally as 'eat medicine'. Its influence is still very strong, and even today many Chinese believe that you should only eat certain foods at certain times of the year. The Chinese are very fond of medicinal soups and other dishes which are suitable for the whole family. Some of these are consumed as special treats, and others only at special times of the year. These are health foods – preventative medicine – and should not be confused with herbal mixtures made up into soup form to treat a specific ailment.

To balance yin and yang, and to improve or restore the flow of qi, herbs are usually taken internally, as a soup or tea, and in combinations of up to twelve individual herbs. Nearly all the herbs used are grown, prepared and packaged in mainland China or Hong Kong, where they are native plants. They also differ in their usage from the herbs of Western herbal medicine: most Chinese herbs are used in a dried or prepared form, whereas most Western herbs are used fresh. Chinese herbs are more similar to Western generic medicines — some even come in the form of pills, ointments or liquid medicines.

Herb combinations

These are based on a variety of factors:

- *Complements* Two or more herbs of similar properties and effects are used together to increase their desired beneficial quality
- *Assistants* Two or more herbs of different properties and effects are used in combination. One herb has the main medicinal effect required, while the other has a catalytic function to increase the effectiveness of the first herb
- *Frights* One herb is used to moderate the action of another, to lessen any dangerous side-effects
- *Hates* One herb is used to modify another's effects so as to achieve the desired result
- *Cancellations* If a herb has inconvenient, though not dangerous, side-effects, a second herb may be used to cancel these out
- *Contrasts* This consists of a mis-combination of two herbs that result in violent bodily reactions, and is rarely pre-scribed

---

Roy

Herbs were combined to treat Roy, a young man of twenty-four who had had a skin complaint since he was fifteen. His skin was itchy, hot and covered with little red spots. Four years earlier he had started work in a plastics factory, and since then his skin had deteriorated considerably. He had a pale red tongue with slight 'white wall'.

His first visit was in June 1993, when he was prescribed a herbal combination of:

Sheng Di Huang *Rehmania glutinosa* (Chinese foxglove root)
Mu Dan Pi *Paeonia suffruticosa* (cortex of tree peony root)
Mu Tong *Akebia trifoliata*
Gan Cao *Glycyrrhiza uralensis* (liquorice root)
Chi Shao *Paeonia veitchii* (red peony root)
Dan Zhu Ye *Lophatherum gracile* (bamboo leaves)
Bai Ji Li *Tribulus terrestris* (caltrop fruit)

He was given three doses and told to return seven days later.

His second visit showed that he was sleeping better, and both the hotness and the red spots had disappeared. There was no itchiness. His tongue was still red, though paler, and the 'white wall' had cleared up.

Roy was given a further six doses to boil and drink every other day in order to stabilize the condition. He was told to return if the condition returned, which to date it has not, and he is considered discharged from the clinic.

OTHER DISCIPLINES IN SUPPORT OF HERBALISM

In China the dividing line between herbalists and practitioners of other disciplines is blurred. A Chinese herbalist may well use acupuncture or moxibustion (see below), while an acupuncturist may well prescribe herbal remedies, perhaps as painkillers. Even a conventional Chinese allopathic doctor may prescribe herbs and/or use acupuncture.

Acupuncture

This technique, which works hand in hand with herbal medicine, was practised in the Stone Age using slivers of stone and bone called *bian*. By around 8000 years BC metal needles were being used; remains of gold acupuncture needles over five thousand years old have been excavated from tombs in Hubei Province.

The qi energy flows along the twelve meridians (see page 24), taking that energy to all parts of the body where it is needed for harmonious health and growth. Sometimes, for various reasons including emotional trauma, infections, poor diet, injury and illness, the meridians become blocked and the qi flow becomes restricted. The whole body can then go into a decline and the original blockage can be difficult to locate. By using metal needles inserted into the meridian lines at specific acupoints the acupuncturist can clear the blockage and reinstate the flow of qi, thus restoring the health of the individual. Over two thousand acupoints have been established but most acupuncturists use on average around 150 (although most treatments would not use more than two or three in any one session).

Moxibustion

Sometimes, when wanting to supplement or tone the energy the acupuncturist will use the technique known as moxibustion, in which a glowing ember of the herb *Artemisia vulgaris* (common mugwort) is used to apply gentle heat to an acupoint. The herb may be burnt in small cones directly on the skin or on the handle of an acupuncture needle to transfer the heat directly into the meridian. The glowing ember is removed as soon as the patient can feel the heat, so there is no risk of being burnt.

Acupressure

If the patient has an aversion to needles, or a fear of the pain that they think they may suffer, or an allergy or blood disorder that would make the insertion of needles inadvisable, then the acupuncturist will apply gentle pressure to the acupoint using their fingers. This is called acupressure, and seems to have the same effect as inserting a needle. It is a treatment especially suitable for children.

Qi gong

In China qi gong is used as a method of preventing illness and promoting good health. Based on a series of physical and meditative exercises that help the flow of qi, it involves some breathing exercises, some martial arts-type movements (it is sometimes used as a martial art in China), and some relaxation and meditation exercises. It is suitable for all age groups and is thought to be especially beneficial to people recovering from illness, as it strengthens qi and quickly restores health. Qi gong is usually practised for about fifteen minutes once a day.

Massage

Chinese medicine practitioners will sometimes decide that the patient's whole body needs to be massaged to restore the flow of qi. Sometimes they will only massage specific points like the shoulders or the back of the neck. It is almost like acupressure, since it moves the qi along the meridians by stimulating the skin and muscles. It is very similar to shiatsu, the Japanese massage technique.

This chapter was intended to be no more than an introductory overview of the herbal aspects of traditional Chinese medicine and other techniques which the practitioner may use in conjunction with herbs. Now let's look more closely at the way a herbalist examines patients, diagnoses what's wrong and arrives at a prescription.

3

How a Chinese Herbalist Diagnoses and Prescribes

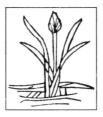

So here you are, having selected your practitioner, arriving for your first consultation. What should you expect?

When you make your first appointment you may well be asked to bring any medical records you have and anything that could be relevant to your complaint. Some people think they can send along a friend or family member to get some medicine on their behalf. But Chinese medicine doesn't work like that — on the first occasion you must go along yourself to be properly examined. If you are too ill to attend the practitioner may, like an ordinary doctor, pay you a house call.

INSIDE THE CLINIC

It will probably look like an old-fashioned Western chemist's shop — the walls will be lined with glass display cases containing a bewildering assortment of potions, lotions, pills and packets. These are imported Chinese generic herbs that can be bought, over the counter, as remedies for coughs and colds, menstrual problems, headaches, upset stomachs and so on — just like the pack of aspirin or bottle of antiseptic mouthwash that you would find in your local chemist. The difference is that the Chinese herbalist's 'pack of aspirin' would contain the herbal equivalent and be packaged more colourfully, with Chinese-style decoration and writing. (A popular brand carries the Tiger logo. This can sometimes cause problems: when herbalists import these products they are often held up by the Customs who suspect they contain parts of real tigers, which are of course a protected species. They don't, but because the ingredients are only listed in Chinese the herbal materials are sometimes sent for analysis.)

Each glass cabinet contains a range of remedies for a particular complaint — one for menstrual and pregnancy problems, another for children's ailments, while yet another might contain remedies for impotence (there is also a Chinese product for over-potency!). Special attention and care are needed in the treatment of pregnant women, since some herbs can induce premature labour or even miscarriage, while others may possibly damage the foetus.

Chinese customers usually know what they want in terms of over-the-counter medication and if they don't they can read the information on the packages. Westerners can't often do that, so they will have to ask. Don't be nervous — the herbalist will be only too happy to help, to give advice and to take time to make sure you have what you need.

Beyond the cabinets of pre-packaged remedies are loose herbs. These are contained in large glass jars or in traditional herbalist's wooden drawers. None of the drawers is marked as the herbalist knows exactly what is in each one. Some of the contents of the jars may look a little strange: that's because not all of them are herbs of the kind you would expect to see, but rather dried remedies of a different kind.

The loose herbs are divided into three categories:

- herbs for healthy eating — for instance adding to soups
- loose herbs bought over the counter instead of the pre-packaged ones
- herbs supplied only on prescription and usually in combinations

When seeds are prescribed, they are usually ground using a mortar and pestle. It is said that you can tell a herbalist from the sound of their mortar and pestle, and their experience and skill can be judged from that sound.

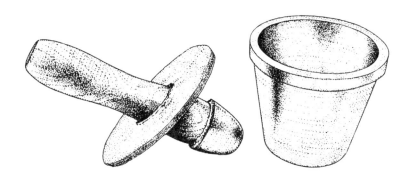

Chinese mortar and pestle

THE CONSULTING ROOM

If it is also used for acupuncture, the consulting room has to be licensed in the UK by the local authority. The licence covers such aspects as hygiene, hand washing facilities and needle sterilization. You should check that a current local authority licence is on display.

There will probably be a couch for acupuncture, and a desk with a chair for you. The walls may display acupuncture charts showing the meridians and acupuncture points of the human body.

THE FOUR EXAMINATIONS (SI JIAN)

Chinese medical practitioners do four vital things:

- *Asking* Finding out the patient's full medical history, their lifestyle, their diet, sex life, fears and upbringing.
- *Looking* Observing the patient's facial colour, general body type and language, the appearance of the tongue, mental state and expression.
- *Listening* Noting the patient's breathing, coughing and voice, and smell (the Chinese regard smell as one of the listening examinations).
- *Feeling* The Chinese practitioner feels for three pulses in each wrist, which indicate the functioning of the major organs, and for the palpation of the flow of qi.

ASKING

Once the herbalist has put you at your ease, found out your name, age and so on, they will want to know about your symptoms and your complaint. They will need to know a lot of information about you — such as your childhood, times of day and year you like best, your medical history and your urine and stool quality, location and type of pain, appetite and tastes, sleep patterns, eating and drinking preferences, and feelings of hot and cold. The herbalist needs all this information because they are not treating the complaint — they are treating you.

Lifestyle (bu nei wai yin)

The Chinese believe very strongly that how a person lives their life affects their health in a very visible way. The ideal is a balanced lifestyle that is in harmony with the universe. This may not seem to be a medical matter, but if your emotions are frayed by an unpleasant situation at work or an unhappy relationship, then your health is bound to be affected. Illness is often a manifestation of some negative quality of life and there may be no cure required beyond change.

Hot and cold

Questions regarding hot and cold point towards identifying the Pernicious Influences and also help characterize yin and yang qualities. Cold generally corresponds to yin and hot to yang for internal disorders. Feeling warm to the touch or disliking heat can point to the External Pernicious Influence of heat or summer heat, while feeling cold to the touch or disliking cold can point to the External Pernicious Influence of cold or dampness.

Pain

The condition of pain is also important, especially when linked to the feelings of hot and cold. Generally, pain lessened by heat signifies cold, while pain lessened by cold signifies heat. Pain with sensations of heaviness signifies dampness; pain moving around signifies wind; superficial pain with tiredness signifies dampness, as does pain which intensifies in humid weather.

Hunger and thirst

These are also important. Thirst is a sign of heat, while lack of thirst indicates cold. Excessive appetite is a sign of the Internal Pernicious Influence of fire, while a low appetite usually signifies dampness.

Diet

The stomach receives food and is responsible for the beginning of the digestive process, and since the spleen is responsible for transforming the food into blood and qi it follows that any disruption or excess of food intake will affect these two organs which in turn will affect the whole body. Too much food taken at one time will not allow the stomach to 'ripen' or the spleen to 'transform'. This leads to stagnant food, which can cause belching, diarrhoea and a distended stomach. Too much raw food strains the yang aspect of the spleen and generates internal cold and internal dampness, causing abdominal pain and diarrhoea. Internal dampness and heat are caused by too much fatty or greasy food and too high an alcohol intake. Sweet foods taken in excess can also cause internal dampness and cold. Insufficient food affects the production of qi and blood, leading to weakness and deficient qi and blood.

Physical activity

There is a balance, as in all things, between too much and too little. With physical activity, and this includes general activities and not just exercise, there is also a time and a season. There is a yang time which includes morning, daytime in general, spring and early summer, and youth. This, when blood and qi are strongest, is the time for active enterprises. There is a yin time which includes evening and night-time in general, autumn and winter, and advancing years. This is the time for quieter activities. In the winter it is suggested that you should go to bed early and get up late, whereas during the summer you should go to bed later and get up earlier. Follow the natural rhythms of life and learn from nature: sleep when you are tired and be active when you are full of energy.

Excessive activity can strain the spleen's ability to manifest qi and blood, leading to a deficiency of these two substances. Excessive idleness can seriously weaken qi and blood. If someone is sluggish and quiet, they may be displaying symptoms of weak qi or blood or causing the qi or blood to become weaker. Someone who is always excessively active could be showing symptoms of hyper-activity or could be draining qi or blood. A practitioner will be able to isolate the cause.

Looking

General appearance

This includes the patient's physical shape, their manner, the way they conduct themselves during the examination and their shen (this is usually translated as spirit or life force). Forceful, talkative people are regarded as yang, whereas quiet, reserved people are usually thought of as yin. Quick movements show heat, while slow movements show cold. Vital, alive eyes indicate strong shen, while dull, cloudy eyes can show a weakened shen. These clues can often help a practitioner make a diagnosis of the condition to be treated.

Facial colour

Ch'i and blood condition can often be determined from the facial colour. In normal healthy people the face should be 'shiny' and 'moist'. If someone is ill but their facial colour is still good this often indicates that the illness is not severe, because the qi and blood are not weakened. Weakened or deficient qi or blood will show in the face as paleness, whereas excess internal heat will make the face glow red. Internal dampness causes a yellow tint, while excessive blackness, especially around the eyes, indicates that there may be a problem affecting the kidneys and that the illness will be chronic and resist treatment.

Tongue

As well as taking the pulses (see page 58), studying the tongue is regarded as one of the most important factors when examining a patient. The tongue is regarded as the only internal organ that can be seen under normal circumstances.

For the purposes of examination the tongue is regarded as having two parts: the tongue itself and the 'fur' that is on it. A normal tongue is pink, indicating good blood flow; the fur should be thin and moist, and the tongue proper should be visible through it.

The size of the tongue will also be considered, as well as its movement and general strength. Each area of the tongue is seen as reflecting the general health of an internal organ: the tip for the lungs, the very tip for the heart, the centre for the spleen and stomach, the sides for the gall bladder and the root for the kidneys.

Fluids

These include phlegm, vomit, sweat and saliva, which the practitioner will examine if necessary. Urine and faeces are classified under 'Asking' as Chinese practitioners rarely request, or examine, specimens in the way that Western doctors do, but rely on a patient's description.

Listening

The practitioner listens to the tone and quality of the patient's voice. Is it strong or does it whine? Is it expressing the facts clearly and forcefully, or does it stammer and sound weak? A loud, clear voice is seen as yang, while a quiet voice is seen as yin. The practitioner will also be listening to see if the voice matches the patient. The patient's cough and breathing will also be listened to.

The smell of a patient, which is included in the listening category, is also important: it can lead to a diagnosis because it indicates the predominant element of the patient. Sometimes the herbalist may even need to taste the patient to confirm a diagnosis. The five elements, smells and tastes are:

- wood/rancid/sour
- fire/scorched/bitter
- earth/fragrant/sweet
- metal/putrid/pungent
- water/rotten/salt

Some of the names may appear rather emotive, but it is just their translation. A Chinese practitioner would mentally use the Chinese equivalents, and not think of someone as 'rotten' or 'rancid'!

Feeling

Apart from actually feeling the skin to ascertain whether the patient feels hot or cold, the practitioner will also 'take the pulses' of the patient. This is the most important aspect of feeling, and is a much more detailed process than pulse-taking in the West. The Chinese practitioner feels for three pulses in each wrist. They do this with the index, middle and third finger of one hand, with their thumb resting lightly across the back of the patient's hand.

Taking the Pulses

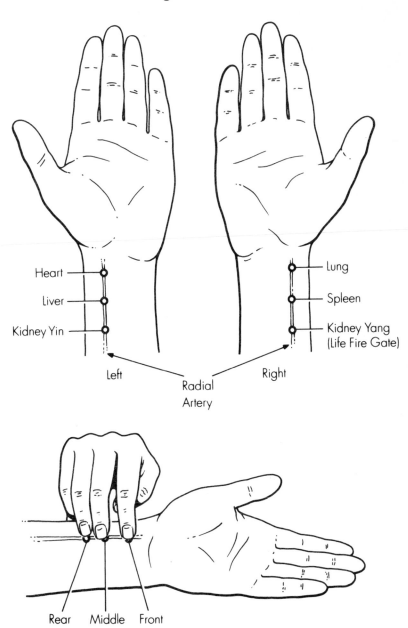

Heart — Liver — Kidney Yin

Lung — Spleen — Kidney Yang (Life Fire Gate)

Left   Right

Radial Artery

Rear   Middle   Front

The pulses are felt for three levels of pressure:

- Deep: quite hard pressure — pushing hard down on to the skin
- Middle: moderate pressure — similar to a Western doctor taking a pulse
- Superficial: light pressure — barely touching the skin

The right wrist
1	First pulse	Lungs
2	Second pulse	Spleen
3	Third pulse	Kidney Yang (Life Fire Gate)

The left wrist
4	First pulse	Heart
5	Second pulse	Liver
6	Third pulse	Kidney Yin

The three pulses at three different pressures in two wrists (18 pulses) are further classified into 28 different types (504 pulse combinations). These are felt for various factors including speed, rhythms, strength, width, quality, shape and length. Given the huge number of combinations Chinese pulse-taking is a very skilled process and takes many years of experience to master.

The 28 combinations

Pulse	Yin/Yang	Significance
Floating (fu mai)	Yang	Deficient yin or Interior wind
Sinking (zhen mai)	Yin	Internal disharmony
Swift (shu mai)	Yang	Heat accelerating the movement of blood

Pulse	Yin/Yang	Significance
Slow (qi mai)	Yin	Cold or insufficient qi
Hollow (kong mai)	Yin	Deficient blood or extreme blood loss
Diffuse (san mai)	Yin	Exhausted kidney yang
Thin (xi mai)	Yin	Deficient qi and/or deficient blood
Large (da mai)	Yang	Excess heat in the stomach
Empty (xu mai)	Yin	Deficient qi and blood
Full (shi mai)	Yang	Excess
Waxy (hua mai)	Yin/yang	Excess of dampness
Choppy (se mai)	Yin	Congealed blood
Moderate (huan mai)	Yin/yang	Normality
Flooding (hong mai)	Yin/yang	Fluids injured by heat
Tiny (wei mai)	Yin	Extreme deficient qi
Frail (ruo mai)	Yin	Deficient qi
Moist (ru mai)	Yin	Deficient blood or internal dampness
Toughened (ge mai)	Yin	Deficient blood
Hidden (fu mai)	Yin	Deficient yang or cold obstructing the meridians
Confined (lao mai)	Yin/yang	Obstruction due to cold
Twisting (dong mai)	Yang	Heart palpitations or extreme fright
Wiry (xuan mai)	Yang	Disharmony of gall bladder and liver
Tight (jin mai)	Yin/yang	Excess cold
Short (duan mai)	Yin	Deficient qi
Long (chang mai)	Yang	Excess qi
Knotted (jie mai)	Yin	Cold obstructing qi
Hurried (cu mai)	Yang	Heat agitating ch'i and blood
Intermittent (dai mai)	Yin	Exhausted organs

DIAGNOSIS BY EXCESSES AND DEFICIENCIES (BIAN ZHENG)

The practitioner will be looking for excesses and deficiencies in four main areas:

- qi
- heat and cold
- yin and yang
- blood

Deficiency	Excess	Symptoms
Qi		Weakness, lethargy, bright pale face, weak pulse, pale tongue, soft voice
	Qi	Localized soreness, swelling, dark or purple tongue, wiry or tight pulse
Heat		Reddish tongue, rapid thin pulse, weakness, slight fever, insomnia, dark urine
	Heat	High fever, rapid or full pulse, constipation, dark meagre urine, delirium, thick yellow fur on tongue, reddish tongue
Cold		Weakness, frailty, abundant clear urine, thin tongue fur, puffy tongue, pulse slow and weak, weak shen
	Cold	Pulse slow and strong, pale tongue, thick white tongue fur, slow movements, clear insufficient urine, cold limbs
Yin		Dizziness, impaired vision, numb limbs, thin body, thin pulse, pale face, dry skin, dry hair, trembling limbs

Deficiency	Excess	Symptoms
	Yin	Pulse slow and strong, pale tongue, thick white tongue fur, slow movements, clear insufficient urine, cold limbs
Yang		Weakness, frailty, abundant clear urine, thin tongue fur, puffy tongue, pulse slow and weak, weak shen
	Yang	High fever, rapid or full pulse, constipation, dark meagre urine, delirium, thick yellow fur on tongue, reddish tongue
Blood		Dizziness, impaired vision, numb limbs, thin body, thin pulse, pale face, dry skin, dry hair, trembling limbs.
	Blood	Blood in urine/vomit/phlegm/faeces, thirst, rapid pulse, irritability, scarlet tongue, delirium

The symptoms for excess cold and excess yin are identical, as are those of deficient yin/deficient blood, deficient cold/deficient yang, excess yang/excess heat. As well as the excesses and deficiencies mentioned, there can also be excesses and deficiencies of all the major organs, as well as the Pernicious Influences. The basic formulae are:

- yin = interior/deficient/cold
- yang = exterior/excess/hot
- yin = weak/pale/thin
- yang = strong/dark/thick

The way a herbalist will use all or some of this information can be seen from the following case history.

Annie

After suffering from migraine for twenty-seven years, and trying every cure known to Western medicine, Annie came to the clinic for help. Her symptoms were intense migraine attacks with pain moving from right to left across her foreheard. For the previous five years she had also suffered from high blood pressure.

She was first seen in December 1992 and diagnosed as having excess liver qi stagnation, with weakness in the stomach and an imbalance between stomach and liver. She was prescribed a herbal remedy of Ju Hua *Chrysanthemum morifolium* (chrysanthemum flowers) and Ju Ming Zi *Cassia tora* (foetid cassia seeds), which is a traditional remedy for migraine. She was given seven doses and a further appointment was made for her in four weeks' time.

At her second appointment, in January 1993, she reported that she had only had one slight migraine during the previous month. She was given a repeat prescription of six doses and told to come again only when, or if, the migraine returned.

She telephoned and made a third visit in June 1993, as she had had further migraine attacks that month. She was given the same prescription and supplied with seven doses.

She didn't return until September 1993 after having a couple more migraines — the first since June. Again she was given the same prescription of seven doses of *Chrysanthemum morifolum* and *cassia tora*.

In December 1993 she telephoned to make sure it was all right if she didn't come back, and was only taking the occasional dose if and when she got a migraine attack. She was assured that that was fine, and hasn't been back since. She put in a repeat prescription for seven doses in May 1994, so had obviously been suffering some recurring symptoms despite her assurances that everything was fine. However, she is now basically considered free of her migraines.

There are two other classifications that may be looked for:

Congealed blood

Haemorrhaging, tumours and lumps, a dark face, a dark purple tongue with red spots, and a choppy pulse indicate this problem.

Stagnant qi

Usually from emotional or dietary causes, qi can get stuck in a particular meridian or organ. The symptoms are swellings and soreness, a dark or purple tongue, and a wiry or tight pulse.

ORGANS AND DIAGNOSIS

Liver and gall bladder

The liver controls the movement of energy throughout the body. Excess yang in the liver results in severe headaches, red and painful eyes and hearing disorders. A disordered liver can result in blood being vomited. Blurred eyesight may be a sign of liver disease. Healthy liver blood can be seen in the fingernails; if they are red and healthy, so is the liver blood.

In Chinese medicine the gall bladder and liver are treated as one organ. A disordered gall bladder may result in bitter gall juices being vomited.

Lungs and large intestine

The lungs are the master of the distribution of qi, and when disordered result in asthma, shortness of breath, a low weak voice, a lack of patience, and laziness. The lungs and large intestine are seen as connected, as both are passages. The nose and voice are seen as the external visible signs of lung and large intestine function.

Tony

Twenty-nine-year-old Tony had suffered from recurrent asthma since he was twelve. He had also had an itchy, cracking skin condition on his body since the age of three. He was diagnosed as having excess phlegm produced by a weakness of his spleen and kidneys, and on his first visit in June 1993 he was given a prescription of a herbal combination consisting of:

Gan Cao *Glycyrrhiza uralensis* (liquorice root)
Jin Yin Hua *Lonicera japonica* (honeysuckle flowers)
Fructus canidii
Ye Ju Hua *Chrysanthemum indicum* (wild
    chrysanthemum flowers)

He was given three doses.

His second visit a week later found him much better. The cracks in his skin had disappeared, and for the first time in twenty-six years he was suffering no itchiness. He was given a repeat prescription of five doses.

Tony was told to return if he had any further skin problems or any asthma attacks, which to date he has not. He was also told that his diet needed looking at (as he was living mainly on 'junk food' with little in the

---

way of fresh fruit and vegetables) and a cream with the same ingredients was recommended if he needed it. He was then considered discharged.

Heart and small intestine

The tongue and the colour of the face are seen as the external visible signs of heart and small intestine function. Impaired heart function can also be detected by loss of memory, fear, nervousness and abnormal gestures, as well as by pulse condition. If the heart's energy is weakened, the pulse will be weak or lacking in strength; if the energy is uneven, the pulse feels irregular and lacking in rhythm.

Spleen and stomach

The lips are said to be the external visible sign of spleen function. A weakened spleen affects the appetite and causes lack of strength in the hands and feet. It can also cause excessive thinness, and white or pale yellow lips. Stomach disorders can produce toothache.

Thelma

Seventy-four-year-old Thelma was referred to us by her dentist as she had been suffering from severe pain on the right side of her face for over a year. The dentist had been unable to discover any reason for the pain.

When Thelma visited the clinic for the first time, in March 1993, she was treated with acupuncture on acupoints R100, R147 and R148 and a further appointment was made for her in one week's time.

When she came back she reported no pain during the

previous week. She could now brush her teeth again, after a year of not being able to do so. Her facial muscles felt comfortable.

She was given a repeat acupuncture treatment using the same acupoints, and has since had no recurrence of the condition.

Kidneys and bladder

Kidneys, known as Fire at the Gate of Life, are the master of the bones, and the teeth are seen as the 'ends of the bones'. Hearing disorders and constipation can also result from kidney disorders. Excess kidney function can cause sexual over-indulgence and irritability, while deficient kidney function can be responsible for impotency, premature ejaculation and unnatural passivity. Normal kidney function can be determined from the hair, as can the bladder function. Weak, brittle hair or excessively dry or greasy hair all point to abnormal kidney function.

DIAGNOSIS

Armed with all this information, the herbalist can then make a diagnosis. This is done not according to Western medicine but in the Chinese way, which means your complaint will be identified as hot or cold, rising or falling, wet or dry. Chinese medical practitioners, remember, don't see a disease or a complaint as something caught or not avoided, but as an imbalance in the body. Using herbs, acupuncture or massage, they will restore the imbalance and return the person to full health. They will also give advice about diet, lifestyle and environment, to try to ensure that the imbalance doesn't occur again. Your herbalist will be as interested in why you have particular symptoms as in the symptoms themselves.

Common ailments and appropriate Chinese herbal remedies are described in Chapter 5.

PRESCRIBING REMEDIES

Once a diagnosis has been made, your herbalist can decide what remedy will benefit you. Again it is *you* who are the important factor. The remedy must restore your imbalance – not kill or eradicate your complaint. Your Chinese herbalist will not see your complaint as something foreign to you, some alien force that is poisoning you, but rather as a part of you that isn't functioning as well as it might. There is no point in waging war on yourself.

When the herbalist has made the diagnosis and selected the remedy you will be given a prescription. This will be made up in the herbalist's shop, where you pay for it in the normal way. You may well be given a repeat prescription that you can bring back at a later date to obtain further stocks, or it may be that your herbalist will want to see you again after a week or so to see what improvement has taken place.

The practitioner may decide that a 'patent remedy' will suit you, rather than something specially made up. This was the situation in the next case history.

Adrian

Thirty-six-year-old Adrian came to see us because he had been suffering bloodstained bowel movements for the previous three years and had been in hospital for six weeks. He was still under medication and his symptoms had reappeared after eighteen months. He was taking four steroid tablets a day: these were affecting his body build and he felt he was getting fat.

His first visit was in April 1992 when he was prescribed a patent Chinese herbal medicine called Fargelin. The dosage was two tablets, twice a day after meals.

After seven days he returned, to report that the bleeding had reduced. Nevertheless there was no real improvement in his general health. He was prescribed the same remedy.

He returned in May and there had been considerable improvement: no blood in his bowel movements, a loss of weight and a general all-round sense of improving health. He still continues with the medication when required, but is considered discharged.

Quantities prescribed

In the same way that remedies are prescribed according to the patient's individual needs, so the quantities prescribed will also vary from patient to patient. Several factors are involved, including the patient's age, overall health and condition, and whether the complaint is improving or deteriorating. The quantities also vary from prescription to prescription because of the herbs themselves: factors taken into account are the freshness or otherwise of the herbs, their quality generally and their combination. There are nine guidelines for prescription quantities:

- *Health* A normally active healthy person would expect to receive a higher dosage than a thin or frail person who has been ill for some time.
- *Age* Elderly patients and children would expect to receive smaller dosages than adults.

- *Condition* Mild cases of an illness obviously need smaller dosages than a chronic or serious case.
- *Taste* Strong-tasting medicines are prescribed in smaller dosages than those with little or no taste.
- *Combination* The main ingredient in a prescription should be in a larger dosage than the others.
- *Category* Ingredients derived from flowers, leaves or stems will be prescribed in smaller amounts than those from minerals, which are much denser.
- *Method* Boiled herbs are prescribed in much larger quantities than those supplied in pill, tablet or powder form.
- *Season* The dosage of the same herbs will vary according to the season in which they were harvested, prepared or dispensed.
- *Environmental* Where the patient lives and/or works may also affect the dosage.

Medicinal soups, tea drinking and other treatments

Sometimes the herbal practitioner will prescribe a medicinal soup to be prepared at home. The ingredients will be supplied by the herbalist, but the cooking conditions are under your own control, so follow the directions closely. During the boiling process a chemical reaction takes place between the herbs. Care must be taken to follow the directions regarding boiling and simmering, as well as the order in which the herbs are to be added to the pan.

Any directions about not drinking tea while a particular course of herbs or soups is being administered should be followed carefully: tea is regarded by the Chinese as a herb in its own right, and should not be combined with others if the advice is not to do so. China teas, of which there are a great variety, remove nicotine from the body, have a diuretic effect, lower blood sugar and assist weight loss.

Your herbalist may, of course, decided that it is not a herbal remedy that you need but rather acupuncture or massage (see pages 47–8). They may be practitioners themselves; alternatively, they can refer you to a competent, qualified one.

4

Herbs and Their Properties

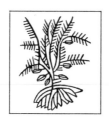

In China the herbs used are gathered from the wild by hand. The best ones grow far from human habitation, and the herbalists who gather them will also be botanists, explorers, climbers and environmentalists. They need to be able to identify the relevant herb in all stages of its development, know where the finest ones grow, be able to get to the plants even when they grow in highly inaccessible places, know how much they can take without threatening a particular species, and always be on the look-out for new sources and new species. Luckily in the West we can just go to our Chinese herbalist's shop and buy them over the counter!

They are mostly imported from Hong Kong, although some come from mainland China via Beijing and Shanghai. Increasingly, as China opens its doors to the West, better access will be granted for importing herbs, but at the time of writing the best stocks are still coming from Hong Kong.

Some herbalists import their herbs directly, while others purchase them from Chinese herbal 'cash and carry' stores in the West or from mail order suppliers (see Useful Addresses).

PRESERVATION

Once the herbs have been collected from the wild they need to be treated so that they will keep their essential qualities during storage. They are always washed and dried. The method of drying varies depending on the particular herb and what it is going to be used for. They may be sun-dried or dried in a clay oven, alone or with other herbs. Sometimes they are dried with minerals such as sulphur, which bleaches them and also acts as a preservative. Occasionally you may hear of herbs being 'treated'. This means that, after drying, they are stir-fried with angelica and milk vetch to enhance their properties. Some may also be buried in the ground to absorb moisture, or cooked in a clay pot with rice wine or honey to increase their potency.

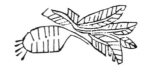

Cutting up herbs

Before or after they have been dried, the herbs will need to be cut up using a herb chopper like the one pictured opposite. When this is done depends on the herb and its eventual usage. There are several ways of cutting herbs. Large roots are often sliced across at 90 degrees, which gives them a round cross-section, while smaller ones are cut at an angle to give a larger surface area. Some herbs are chopped very finely and compressed into a cake.

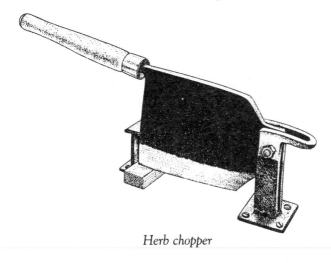

Herb chopper

Some herbs have to be ground to a powder and this is done using a mortar and pestle with a lid, to avoid the loss of powder during crushing.

Storage

Traditionally, herbs would be stored in clay pots after preservation and cutting up. The shape of the clay pots and whether they were covered or uncovered depended on the herbs. The Chinese have always used clay pots, because clay was the simplest and cheapest material to get hold of and also because, when glazed and therefore non-absorbent, it helped to keep the properties of the herbs intact.

Modern herbalists increasingly use glass jars and bottles for herb storage, but still rely on wooden drawers for the bulk of their stocks because this is the easiest and most convenient method of dispensing them. These drawers are rarely labelled, as the herbalist is completely familiar with their contents. Since the drawers are arranged according to meridians and properties it would be hard for the herbalist to make a mistake that would result in a herb of a totally different type being dispensed.

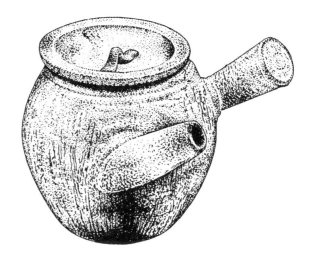

Clay pot

Freshness of stocks

However the herbs are stored, herbalists will check them periodically for mould and other signs of decay. Don't worry about whether these checks will be carried out − any fungal infection is likely to affect an entire stock of herbs, so it's in the herbalist's own best interests to check most of their stocks every day to be on the safe side.

Herbs may need to be retreated − that is, washed and boiled, redried and, where necessary, freshly treated with angelica again in the same way that fresh herbs are.

Weighing herbs

Because it is so expensive, ginseng is weighed in very sensitive scales which have divisions of 0.1 of a gram.

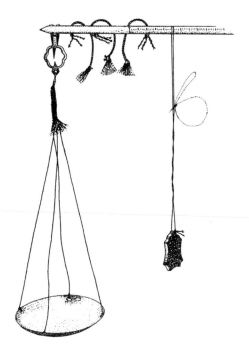

Ginseng scales

Other herbs do not need quite such accurate scales, and larger ones can be used. These are accurate to within approximately 3 grams. Both sorts of scales are used by holding one of the strings near the pan and adjusting the weight on the rod.

Metric weights have been used for convenience throughout this book, but Chinese herbalists use Chinese weights. Their names and metric equivalents are given below.

1 fan		= 0.3 grams approx
10 fan	= 1 qin	= 3 grams approx
10 qin	= 1 lian	= 30 grams approx
16 lian	= 1 jin	= 480 grams approx

Whatever scales are used, the weight given is always that of the herb before any stir frying which may be specified on the prescription. The herbs may be fried in honey, water or rice wine, or 'burned' until black in a red-hot wok. These treatments naturally change the weight of the herb, and it is not unknown for patients to weigh their herbs afterwards and mistakenly complain that they have been short-changed by the herbalist.

Boiling and steaming

As soon as possible after collection, the herbs are boiled in clay pots. These come in a variety of shapes and sizes much like Western saucepans. It used to be traditional to throw away all pots used in medicinal preparations on the Chinese New Year's Eve. But few herbalists in the West can afford to do this now, especially since some of the decorated pots are extremely expensive.

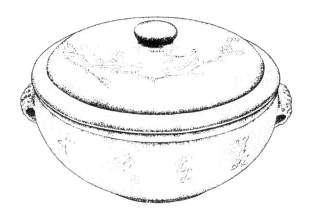

Decorated pot

Steam pots are used a lot for medicinal foods. The ingredients are added to the pot, after which both lids are put on and fastened by a string which passes through the handles. The pot is then placed in a larger pot of boiling water. The herbs and other ingredients are gently cooked by the rising steam without losing any valuable elements which might otherwise be boiled out.

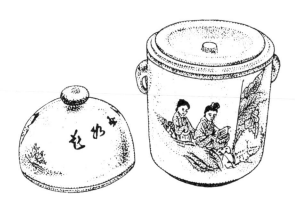

Steam pot

PROPERTIES OF COMMONLY USED CHINESE HERBS

In the following lists the Chinese name has been used, along with the botanical name and the Western common name where possible. (Some Chinese herbs are not native to the West and have no corresponding Western name so in these cases the literal English translation has often been included.) Most of the herbs described in this chapter can be used in their fresh state, but they can all be ordered as dried herbs from any of the importers listed in the Useful Address section. Dosages given are standard ones from which herbalists would raise or lower according to the individual. It is interesting to note that many of the Chinese names have suffixes denoting parts of the plant for example: hua/flower; pi/cortex or peel; ren/seeds; ye/leaf; zi/ fruit or seeds.

Bai Shao *Paeonia lactiflora, P. obovata,* White peony root

Part used: root, sliced.
Meridian: liver.
Taste: sweet.
Usage: for abdominal pains after childbirth combine with Dang Gui (*Angelica sinensis*/Chinese angelica), Chuan Xiong (*Ligustrum wallichii*/Szechuan lovage root) and Hong Hua (*Carthamus tinctorius*/safflower).
Dosage: 6–15 g.
Note: do not use with black false hellebore (*Veratrum nigrum*).

Bai Zhu *Atractylodes macrocephala* Atractylodes

Part used: root.
Meridians: spleen, stomach.
Taste: bitter-sweet.
Usage: to correct mischannelling of qi at the spleen and stomach. Used to treat loss of appetite, extended tight abdomen, vomiting and bowel disorders. It is safe to use during pregnancy.
Dosage: 4.5–9 g.

Gan Cao *Glycyrrhiza uralensis, G. glabra* Liquorice

Part used: root.
Meridians: all.
Taste: sweet.
Usage: one of the most frequently used Chinese herbs. It can be used on its own to assist the spleen, dispel heat and restore qi. It is used to treat sore throats and to relieve food poisoning.

It is most often used with other herbs to moderate their effects. It is also used to alleviate any uncomfortable side-effects which may be felt after taking other medicinal herbs.
Dosage: 1.5–9 g.

Gou Qi Zi *Lycium chinense* Lycium

Part used: seed.
Meridians: liver, kidneys.
Taste: sweet.
Usage: to strengthen shen and kidneys, and to improve eyesight, used with Sheng Di Huang (*Rehmania glutinosa*/ Chinese foxglove root), Ju Hua (*Chrysanthemum morifolium*/ chrysanthemum) and Shan Zhu Yu (*Cornus officinalis*/fruit of Asiatic cornelian cherry). Used with Sheng Di Huang (*Rehmania glutinosa*) and Tian Men Dong (*Asparagus cochinchinensis*/asparagus root) to treat deficient liver and/or kidneys as well as tinnitus, dizziness and weakness of the knees, and for the prevention of wet dreams.
Dosage: 6–12 g.

Gou Teng *Nauclea rhyncholphylla* (also *Unicaria*)

Part used: thorn.
Meridians: heart, liver.
Taste: sweet.
Usage: to stop convulsions, tics and spasms used with Tian Ma (*Gastrodia elata*/Gastrodia rhizome). For the treatment of red eyes caused by headaches used with Ju Hua (*Chrysanthemum morifolium*/chrysanthemum), Sang Ye (*Morus alba*/white mulberry leaves) and Bo He (*Mentha arvensis*/mint). It does not need boiling.
Dosage: 6–12 g.

Gui Zhi *Cinnamomum cassia* Cinnamon twigs

Part used: bark.
Meridians: heart, lungs, bladder.
Taste: sweet.
Usage: used in combination with Ma Huang (*Ephedra sinica/* Ephedra) if the patient does not sweat; if they do, given with peeled Chi Shao (*Paeonia veitchii/*red peony root). Used in combination with Qiang Huo (*Notopterygium incisum*) to relieve pain in joints, especially arthritis. Used with Dang Gui (*Angelica sinensis/*Chinese angelica) or Chuan Xiong (*Ligustrum wallichii/* Szechuan lovage root) to treat period pains and menstrual irregularity.
Dosage: 3–9 g (slightly more if used for arthritis).
Note: avoid during pregnancy.

Huang Qi *Astragalus membranaceus* Milk vetch

Part used: root, sliced, either raw or stir-fried in honey.
Meridians: lungs, spleen.
Taste: sweet.
Usage: given as a tonic to patients recovering from illness or feeling tired and weak. Can be used in conjunction with ginseng. This is one of most commonly prescribed herbs in Chinese medicine, and symptoms which would point to its use include loss of appetite, coldness, shortness of breath and a tendency to sweat a lot.
Dosage: 9–30 g.

Huang Qin *Scutellaria baicalensis* Baical skullcap root

Part used: root, raw or stir-fried in rice wine.
Meridians: gall bladder, small intestine, lungs, large intestine, spleen.
Taste: bitter.

Usage: for throat pain used with Lian Qiao (*Forsythia suspensa/* forsythia fruit) and Jin Yin Hua (*Lonicera japonica/*honeysuckle flower). For relieving high blood pressure used with Ju Hua (*Chrysanthemum morifolium/*chrysanthemum) and Gou Teng *Nauclea rhyncholphylla.*

Dosage: 3–10 g.

Jing Jie   *Schizonepeta tenuifolia*

Part used: seeds.
Meridians: none specific.
Taste: tangy.
Usage: to stop swellings and as an excellent painkiller. Used more than any other herb for the treatment of arthritis. Fried until very dark in colour it is used to stop bleeding, especially from haemorrhoids.
Dosage: 3–9 g.

Ma Huang   *Ephedra sinica*   Ephedra

Part used: stalk.
Meridians: bladder, lungs.
Taste: tangy.
Usage: used in combination with Gui Zhi (*Cinnamomum cassia/*cinnamon) to aid sweating. Stir-fried in honey and apricot kernels, restores the function of the lungs and suppresses asthma, especially with coughing. Used with Sheng Jiang (*Zingiber officinale/*fresh ginger rhizome (root) and Bai Zhu (*Atractylodes macrocephala*) to reduce swelling.
Dosage: 3–9 g.
Note: not suitable for patients who suffer from insomnia or high blood pressure. Not to be used by patients who are already sweating.

Mai Men Dong   *Ophiopogon japonicus*   'Lush winter wheat'

Part used: root nodules, used raw and pressed flat.
Meridians: stomach, lungs, heart.
Taste: bitter.
Usage: to restore yin. Used with Ban Xia (*Pinellia ternata*/'Half summer') and liquorice for coughs and dry throat. Used with Sheng Di Huang (*Rehmania glutinosa*/Chinese foxglove root), Xuan Shen (*Scrophularia ningpoensis*/Ningpo figwort root), Huang Lian (*Coptis chinensis*/golden thread) and Dan Shen (*Salvia miltiorrhiza*/'Scarlet root') for insomnia.
Dosage: 6–12 g.

Mu Dan Pi   *Paeonia suffruticosa*   Tree peony

Part used: bark.
Meridians: kidneys, liver, heart.
Taste: bitter.
Usage: to lower high blood pressure, used with Ju Hua (*Chrysanthemum morifolium*/chrysanthemum) and Jin Yin Hua (*Lonicera japonica*/honeysuckle flower). For menstrual disorders, used with Chai Hu (*Bupleurum chinense*/thorowax) and Dang Gui (*Angelica sinensis*/Chinese angelica). To stop bleeding in internal wounds, dry-fried until dark and given with Hong Hua (*Carthamus tinctorius*/safflower). For period pain, raw slices given with Gui Zhi (*Cinnamomum cassia*/cinnamon) and Hu Tao Ren (*Juglans regia*/walnut). To stimulate the production of blood and to disperse bruises, used fried in rice wine with cinnamon and walnuts.
Dosage: 6–12 g.
Note: not suitable for use during pregnancy.

Qing Hao   *Artemisia annua, A. apiacea*   Wormwood

Part used: leaves.
Meridians: liver, gall bladder.

Taste: bitter, but with a very pleasant smell.

Usage: for the treatment of burns and minor skin disorders, fresh leaves are crushed and applied externally. For the treatment of malaria, used with Huang Qin (*Scutellaria baicalensis*/Baical skullcap root). Ban Xia (*Pinellia ternata*) and *Maronta arundinacea* (arrowroot).

Dosage: 20–40 g for malaria, 6–15 g for skin application.

Note: this herb responds best to rapid, short boiling.

San Qi   *Panax notoginseng*   Pseudoginseng root

Part used: whole plant (it is similar to ginseng).

Meridians: kidneys, liver.

Taste: bitter.

Usage: to disperse bruises, relieve swellings and stop haemorrhaging, and for general relief of pain.

Dosage: for wounds and pain 1–1.5 g powder three times a day; for cardiac arrest 1.5 g twice a day in equal proportions with ginseng.

Shan Zhu Yu   *Cornus officinalis*   Cornelian Asiastic cherry

Part used: flesh of fruit.

Meridians: liver, kidneys.

Taste: bitter-sour.

Usage: used in the treatment of abnormally heavy menstruation. Used with ginseng to treat heavy sweating accompanied by exhaustion.

Dosage: 4.5–9 g.

Shi Chang Pu   *Acorius gramineus*   Sweetflag

Part used: root.

Meridians: heart, spleen, stomach.

Taste: tangy.

Usage: for excess tan (mucus). Used with Zhi Zi (*Gardenia jasminoides*/Cape jasmine), young bamboo leaves and extracted ginger juice for treating delirium. To treat tinnitus and amnesia, given with Fu Ling (*Poria cocos*/hoelen) and Yuan Zhi (*Polygala tenuifolia*/root of Chinese Senega). For loss of appetite, given with Huo Xiang (*Agastache rugosa*/Patchouli), Huo Po (*Magnolia officinalis*/magnolia) and Chen Pi (*Citrus reticulata*/tangerine peel).
Dosage: 3–9 g.

Shu Di Huang *Rehmania glutinosa* Root of Chinese foxglove cooked in wine

Part used: root (oven dried or fresh).
Meridians: liver, kidneys, heart.
Taste: sweet.
Usage: (a) to relieve cold in the blood. Used with Xuan Shen (*Scrophularia ningpoensis*/Ningpo figwort) to reduce high body temperature, dry mouth and red tongue. Given with He Ye (*Nelumbo necifera*/lotus leaves) and Qian Cao Gen (*Rubia cordifolia*/Madder root) for blood in vomit or urine. Used with Mu Dan Pi (*Paeonia suffruticosa*/cortex of tree peony root) for macula or dark spots on the skin. To treat thirst associated with diabetes, used with Bi Xie Xu Duan (*Dioscorea batatas*/Chinese yam) and Di Gu Pi (*Lycium chinense*/Chinese wolfberry).
(b) Used dried, then fried in rice wine until dark, for restoration of the blood, weakness of the knees, menstrual disorders and tinnitus.
Dosage : (a) 9–30 g (double if fresh), (b) 9–15 g.

Tian Ma *Gastrodia elata* Gastrodia rhizome

Part used: tuber.
Meridian: liver.
Taste: sweet.

Usage: to clear collateral channels and to relieve rheumatic pain, given with Jin Yin Hua (*Lonicera japonica*/honeysuckle flower) and Huai Niu Xi (*Achyranthes bidentata*/'Ox knee'). Given with Ban Xia (*Pinellia ternata*/'Half summer') and Bai Zhu (*Atractylodes macrocephala*) in the treatment of migraine, eye disorders and dizziness. Excellent for women suffering headaches, especially after childbirth.

Dosage: 3–9 g boiled in water, 1–1.5 g as a powder.

Tian Men Dong *Asparagus cochinchinensis* Tuber of Chinese asparagus

Part used: root, raw and sliced.
Meridians: lungs, kidneys.
Taste: bitter-sweet.
Purpose: to restore deficient yin. Dispels heat and strengthens the kidneys and lungs.
Usage: to treat a dry cough with little mucus, or coughing up of blood, use with Mai Men Dong (*Ophiopogon japonicus*/'Lush winter wheat') and Bei Mu (*Fritillaria verticillata*/fritillaria bulb). For use in the treatment of whooping cough with Mai Men Dong (*Ophiopogon japonicus*/'Lush winter wheat') and Bai Bu (*Stemona sessilifolia*/stemona root).
Dosage: 6–12 g.

Tu Si Zi *Cuscuta chinensis* Dodder seeds

Part used: seeds, boiled and crushed, sometimes in cake form.
Meridians: kidneys, lungs.
Taste: sweet.
Purpose: to treat deficient yang in the kidneys, which causes frequent urination. Also used to prevent miscarriages and to help restore the function of the kidneys and menstrual cycle.
Dosage: 6–12 g.

Wu Wei Zi *Schizandra chinensis, S. sphenanthera* Schisandra fruit

The Chinese name means 'the fruit which has five tastes'. It has two forms, northern (*S. chinensis*) and southern (*S. sphenanthera*).

Part used: fruit, raw or steamed with vinegar or rice wine.
Meridians: kidneys, heart, lungs.
Taste: sour.
Usage: for coughs caused by weakness of the lungs, sometimes in combination with ginseng. Use with Mai Men Dong (*Ophiopogon japonicus*/'Lush winter wheat') to treat patients who sweat, have a dry mouth, tire easily and are depressed.
Dosage: 1.5–6 g.

Xin Yi Hua *Magnolia liliflora* Magnolia flower

Part used: flower.
Meridians: none specific.
Taste: tangy.
Usage: for the treatment of rhinitis and nasosinusitis. Clears running nose and headaches.
Dosage: 1–3 g.

Yin Yang Huo *Epimedium brevicornum, E. grandiflorum, E. sagittatum* 'Licentious goat wort'

Part used: the whole plant apart from the root.
Meridians: liver, kidneys.
Taste: sweet.
Usage: used to treat high blood pressure in elderly women, impotence and paralysis of the lower limbs.
Dosage: 3–9 g.

Yu Xing Cao *Houttuynia cordata* 'Fishy smelling herb'

Part used: whole herb.
Meridians: kidneys, lungs.
Taste: sweet with a fishy odour, hence it is also known as the smelly fish plant.
Usage: the treatment of lung and kidney disorders.
Dosage: 9–30 g.

Yuan Zhi *Polygala tenuifolia* Root of Chinese senega

Part used: root, chopped and treated with liquorice.
Meridians: lungs, heart, kidneys.
Taste: bitter.
Usage: for treatment of irritability, insomnia and depression.
Dosage: 3–9 g.

Zi Su Ye *Perilla frutescens* Perilla leaf

Part used: leaves.
Meridians: spleen, lungs.
Taste: sweet.
Usage: to promote ch'i, to relieve pain and tightness in the abdomen, to cancel out the effects of food poisoning (especially when caused by seafood), to ease vomiting and diarrhoea.
Dosage: 6–12 g.

Also part of the herbalist's traditional repertoire will be such well-known herbs as ginseng, garlic and ginger. Ginseng (*Panax ginseng*) is the dried root of the Ren Shen plant which is grown mainly in Japan and Korea. Its main uses are to help strengthen weak bodies and to help patients recovering after illness. It is used extensively as a nutritive and restorative tonic and to treat impotence, neurasthenia, spermatorrhea, anaemia, senility, uterine disorders and nephritis.

Ginger is the fresh root of *Zingiber officianale* (Gan Jiang) and is used mainly as as stomach restorative. It is used in the treatment of nausea and vomiting as well as diarrhoea, rheumatism, abdominal and spleen ache and sometimes for strider—obstructed breathing.

Garlic (*Allium sativum*) known as Xie Bai to the Chinese, is used to 'thin the blood'. It is known to reduce blood cholesterol, prevent heart disease, aid digestion and to lower blood pressure.

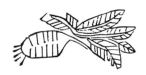

5

Common Ailments and Their Treatment with Chinese Herbal Medicine

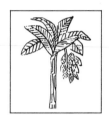

As Chinese herbal medicine is a holistic system based on the individual needs of the patient, it is difficult to prescribe treatment in a book. Each patient and each illness is unique. If two people are suffering from the same condition, it is unlikely that each will receive the same remedy. Self-diagnosis is not recommended; however, basic remedies can be used for mild conditions that would normally be treated at home. If you are in any doubt, go to a trained and qualified practitioner.

All the made-up remedies and recipe ingredients can be obtained from the stockists listed at the back of the book. For convenience, only common plant names have been used in this chapter; see the glossary for their Chinese and botanical equivalents.

Abscesses

Source: heat and fire poison in the blood.
Use: (internal) a tea made from violet, wild chrysanthemum or dandelion, and golden thread; (external) peony flowers or rhubarb crushed and mixed with vegetable oil as ointment.

Acid Stomach

Source: deficient spleen, imbalance of liver and spleen.
Treatment: tonify spleen, dry dampness, soothe the liver, reduce stagnation.
Use: ginseng, liquorice, tangerine peel. Avoid cold food, acidic food.

Alcoholism

Source: excess heat.
Treatment: clear heat from blood and liver.
Use: watermelon or kudzu vine to detoxify blood.

Amnesia

Source: kidney weakness.
Treatment: strengthen kidney weakness.
Use: wolfberry seed, mulberry fruit, eucommia bark, dodder seed.

Anaemia

Source: spleen not transforming qi properly.
Use: Gui Pi Wan (Return Spleen Tablets).

Angina

Source: stagnating qi in blood and heart.
Use: safflower, cinnamon twigs, red sage root, peony root, macrosten onion bulb.
Note: this condition is serious and should not be treated at home. Consult a qualified practitioner.

Anorexia

Source: weakness of stomach and spleen.
Use: wheat sprouts, rice sprouts, loganberries, radish seeds.

Anxiety

Source: weakness of spleen, depression of liver qi.
Treatment: strengthen spleen and enliven liver qi.
Use: ginseng, Chinese angelica. White peony root with thorowax root for relaxation.

Arthritis (see also Rheumatoid Arthritis)

Source: wind damp. Painful joints are caused by wind cold.
Use: cinnamon twigs to release qi, aconite root, angelica root and wild ginger to relieve cold and damp.
Note: if there are not painful joints it is regarded as wind heat, because the joints are usually swollen and hot. Use large-leaved gentian and cork tree bark.

Asthma

Source: phlegm produced by weakness of spleen and kidneys.
Use: almond and ephedra to open up lung passages.
Note: there are many causes of asthma. Seek qualified diagnosis.

Back Pain

Source: too many to list, including physical injury.
Treatment: acupuncture, massage, qi gong.
Use: teasel root, ginseng and acanthopanax root to relieve pain.

Bedwetting

Source: weak kidney qi.
Use: walnut and black ginger seeds to tonify the kidneys.

Blood Pressure: High

Source: regarded as internal wind.
Treatment: calm liver yin and blood wind.
Use: peony root, chrysanthemum flowers and astralagus.

Blood Pressure: Low

Source: regarded as deficient qi in blood and the heart.
Use: ginseng and Chinese angelica.

Bronchitis

Source: (acute) external wind, cold or heat; (chronic) internal deficient spleen or lungs, or internal mucus.
Use: (acute) fritillary bulb, plantain seed and balloon flower root; (chronic) honeysuckle flowers, mulberry leaves and gardenia fruit.

Cancer

Source: deficient qi, deficient blood or deficient yin or yang.
Treatment: consult qualified practitioner.

Cataracts

Source: weak liver and kidneys due to deficient blood.
Use: wolfberry, chrysanthemum flowers, rumania and dendronbrum.

Catarrh

Sources: many.
Use: blackberry leaves, peppermint and magnolia flowers. Use ginger and orange peel in food.

Chickenpox (see also Shingles)

Source: wind and heat invasion.
Use: safflower, cimicifuga and honeysuckle.

Chilblains

Source: deficient yang qi.
Use: cinnamon twigs, red sage, angelica, dried ginger and aconite root.

Chills

Source: external cold (can be symptom of onset of more serious condition).
Use: ginger.

Colon, Spastic (see Spastic Colon)

Conjunctivitis

Source: wind heat in liver meridians.
Use: boil bamboo leaves, violets and chrysanthemum flowers and use the water to bathe eyes.

Cystitis

Source: damp heat.
Use: plantain seeds.

Deafness

Source: many, including physical injury.
Treatment: consult practitioner.

Depression

Source: stagnation of liver qi.
Use: angelica, peony root, liquorice and thorowax root.

Diabetes

Source: sweet urine disease, yin, deficient heat, lung disorder.
Use: to help nourish spleen, kidneys and stomach use Chinese yam, lotus seed and mulberry.
Note: Insulin-dependent diabetics must see a practitioner before administering any self-remedy.

Diarrhoea

Source: many and varied.
Use: (acute) skullcap root, golden thread, kapok flowers and dandelion root; (chronic) psoralea fruit, codonopsis root and astragalus.

Dizziness

Source: (chronic) kidney deficient, or liver heat in cases of high blood pressure; (acute) wind invasion in cases after illness such as influenza.
Use: fresh ginger, cinnamon twigs and peppermint. For nourishing blood, use mulberry.

Dysentery

Source: damp heat external.
Use: peony root, skullcap root, golden thread and anemone.

Eczema

Source: (open weeping). damp heat, (dry red) excess heat in blood; (allergic) wind.
Use: for allergic eczema use ledebouriella root and schizonepeta or peony root, Chinese gentian and rumania. See practitioner for the other types.

Epilepsy

Source: excess heart mucus, internal damp, stagnant qi or blood.
Treatment: consult a practitioner.
Use: sweet flag root and the juice from young bamboo can sometimes cut down the number of attacks.

Exhaustion

Source: deficient qi or blood.
Use: ginseng and astragalus.

Eyesight (to restore or improve tired eyes)

Source: exhausted blood.
Use: wolfberry, mulberry, chrysanthemum flowers and cassia seed.

Flatulence

Source: stagnant stomach qi or damp heat.
Use: orange peel, perilla stem and magnolia bark.

Flu

Source: wind cold, damp, wind heat.
Treatment: moxibustion.
Use: honeysuckle, peppermint, chrysanthemum and cinnamon.

Frozen Shoulder

Source: weak yang qi, external cold and damp.
Treatment: acupuncture.
Use: cinnamon twigs and turmeric.

German Measles (see Rubella)

Hair Loss

Source: deficient liver and kidneys.
Use: wolfberry, mulberry and fleece flower root.

Halitosis

Source: stomach damp heat.
Use: golden thread, peppermint tea, giant hyssop and radish seeds.

Hepatitis A

Source: (acute) excess liver and gall bladder damp heat.
Treatment: consult practitioner.
Use: gardenia fruit and Oriental wormwood.

Hepatitis B

Source: (viral) deficient qi, weakened liver.
Treatment: consult a practitioner.
Use: peony root, mulberry, ginseng, liquorice and astragalus.

Hiccups

Source: heat, cold or food stagnation.
Use: berilla stems, rhubarb and ginger.

Impotence

Source: weakness of kidneys and liver, liver qi stagnation.
Use: cibot root.

Incontinence

Source: kidney yang deficiency with internal cold.
Use: Golden Lock Tea.

Indigestion

Source: weakness of spleen and stomach.
Use: rice and wheat sprouts.

Infertility

Source: damp heat, imbalance of yin and yang.
Treatment: consult practitioner.

Insomnia

Source: heat in heart driving out shen, weakness in kidneys, over-eating.
Treatment: massage, acupressure and exercise.
Use: hoelen, fleece flower stem and wild jujube. Sleep on a gypsum pillow.

Irritable Bowel Syndrome

Source: weakness of kidneys and spleen, excess dampness in intestines, liver qi stagnation.
Use: dandelion, rhubarb, magnolia and angelica.

Itching

Source: external or internal wind.
Use: dittany bark, puncture vine fruit.

Jaundice

Source: dampness in gall bladder and liver.
Treatment: consult a practitioner.
Use: gardenia fruit, Oriental wormwood and cork tree bark.

Laryngitis

Source: poisoned heat in lungs.
Use: peppermint, honeysuckle flowers, mulberry, lily and liquorice.

Ligaments (Torn and Sprained)

Source: internal blood and qi stagnation.
Treatment: acupuncture, massage and herbal plasters.
Use: safflower, ginseng and millettia stem.

Lumbago

Source: many, including physical injury and excess internal cold.
Use: tincture of achyranthes root and acanthopanax bark in alcohol.

Malaria

Source: internal and external simultaneously (see Pernicious Influences).
Use: Bupleurum Tonic and Seven Wonder Tonic. It could well be necessary to add or subtract ingredients.

Mastitis

Source: stagnant qi and blood.
Use: peony bark, dandelion, Chinese gentian and madder root.

ME (Myalgic Encephalomyelitis)

Source: weakness of qi, deficient blood, damp heat.
Treatment: responds well to acupuncture.

Measles (see also Rubella)

Source: excess heat in blood and stomach.
Use: peppermint, safflower and honeysuckle.

Memory Loss

Source: deficient kidney essence.
Use: dodder seeds, mulberry and black ginger seed.

Menopause (to alleviate symptoms such as hot flushes)

Source: weakness of kidneys, deficient blood and imbalance between kidney and liver.
Use: angelica, peony root and thorowax root.

Menstrual Problems

Source: (excessive flow) heat in blood; (scanty flow) cold in blood; (late periods) cold in blood; (painful periods) cold in blood.
Treatment: acupuncture, moxibustion.

Migraine

Source: excess liver qi stagnation, weakness in stomach, imbalance of stomach and liver.
Treatment: acupuncture; consult a practitioner.
Use: chrysanthemum, cassia tora.

Morning Sickness

Source: excess cold, weakness of stomach.
Use: fresh ginger, ginger tea. Avoid cold foods.

Mosquito Bites

Source: poisoned blood.
Use: palm oil applied externally.

Mumps

Source: wind, damp heat.
Use: dandelion, honeysuckle, skullcap and rhubarb.

Nausea

Source: ascending stomach qi.
Treatment: acupressure.

Nephritis

Source: Heat invading lung, weakness of spleen, deficient kidneys.
Treatment: consult practitioner.

Nettle Rash

Source: heat and wind when red and hot, cold and wind when a cold white rash.
Use: schizomeotea, ledebouriella.

Neuritis

Source: wind, damp and heat invading meridians.
Treatment: consult practitioner.

Nose and Throat Conditions

Source: weakness of lung, cold and wind.
Use: plantain seed, peppermint, mulberry, honeysuckle and skullcap.

Nosebleed

Source: heat in blood.
Use: peony root, thistle, rumania.

Obesity

Source: excess mucus and dampness, weakened spleen.
Treatment: acupuncture, exercise, qi gong. Consult a practitioner.

Oedema

Source: excess water, kidney deficiency.
Use: ginseng, water plantain, poria, cinnamon twigs, ephedra.

Osteoarthritis

Source: weakness in kidneys, blood stagnation.
Use: ledebouriella root, cinnamon twigs, tinospora stem, angelica. Avoid cold.

Osteoporosis

Source: kidney deficiency.
Use: cibot rhizome, drynaria tuber, eucommia bark.

Palpitations

Source: heart blood deficiency.
Treatment: acupuncture.
Use: asparagus root, wild jujube seed.

Parkinson's Disease

Source: deficient blood, deficient kidney yin.
Treatment: acupuncture.
Use: gastrodia tuber, peony root, peony buds, wolfberry root.

Peptic Ulcer

Source: stagnating stomach qi, weakness of spleen, excess heat.
Use: ginseng, dandelion, corydalis tuber. Avoid cold food, alcohol, coffee, tea.

Phlebitis

Source: excess heat in blood.
Use: golden thread, peony bark, safflower, rhubarb root.

PMS (Premenstrual Syndrome)

Source: imbalance of spleen, kidneys and liver.
Use: angelica, skullcap, hoelen, peony.

Pneumonia

Source: mucus and heat in lung(s).
Treatment: consult a practitioner.
Use: peach kernel, skullcap, fritillary bulb.

Poliomyelitis

Source: weak qi and blood.
Treatment: consult a practitioner. Acupuncture.

Prolapse (of any organ)

Source: deficient qi.
Use: Central Qi Pills.

Prostate Problems

Source: excess dampness, stagnant qi.
Use: cinnamon bark, cork tree bark, water plantain.

Quinsy (Suppurative Tonsillitis)

Source: fire and heat poison in blood.
Use: golden thread, dandelion, skullcap, forsythia fruit.

Restlessness

Source: yin or blood deficiency.
Use: lotus seed sprouts and felskrone root made into a tea.

Rheumatism

Source: qi stagnation, excess wind, damp and heat.
Use: achyranthus root ('Ox knee') and cork tree bark.

Rheumatoid Arthritis (see also Arthritis)

Source: excess internal coldness.
Treatment: acupuncture.
Use: powdered rhubarb and sesame oil.

Rubella (German Measles)

Source: external wind, heat.
Use: mulberry, honeysuckle, chrysanthemum.

Sciatica

Source: heat stagnation in gall bladder.
Treatment: acupuncture.

Scrofula

Source: liver and kidney yin deficiency.
Use: gardenia fruit, fritillary bulb, eclipta.

Seasickness

Source: external movement.
Use: fresh ginger.

Shingles (see also Chickenpox)

Source: gall bladder heat and damp.
Use: gentian and Oriental wormwood.

Sinusitis

Source: deficient lung qi.
Use: honeysuckle, peppermint, fritillary bulb.

Spastic Colon

Source: excess cold, stagnant qi, weak blood.
Use: fresh ginger, cinnamon twigs, peony, astragalus.

Spots and Pimples

Source: excess heat in blood and stomach.
Use: herbal teas of chrysanthemum, dandelion and honeysuckle. Apply cucumber and watermelon juice.

Sweating

Source: qi deficiency, yin deficiency.
Use: (qi deficiency) ledebouriella and astragalus; (yin deficiency) lilyturf root, cork tree bark and peony.

Tennis Elbow

Source: cold and damp in elbow.
Use: mulberry twigs, cinnamon twigs, angelica root and ginger.

Thrush

Source: excess damp, damp heat.
Use: gentian and Oriental wormwood.

Tonsillitis

Source: fire, poison, wind and heat.
Use: honeysuckle tea. Avoid spicy food.

Toothache

Source: heat in stomach, decayed or damaged teeth.
Treatment: acupuncture; visit a dentist.
Use: gypsum to relieve heat, ginseng.

Ulcer, Peptic (see Peptic Ulcer)

Ulcerated Colitis

Source: poisoned blood, excess damp.
Use: dandelion, astragalus.

Varicose Veins

Source: bad circulation, stagnant qi, stagnant blood.
Use: (internally) angelica, cinnamon twigs, astragalus, (externally) honey.

Vertigo

Source: blood deficiency, qi deficiency, liver wind.
Treatment: consult a practitioner.

6

Prescriptions
and Medicinal Foods

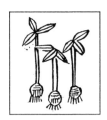

The way Chinese herbal practitioners classify ailments is somewhat different from that of their Western counterparts. As their fundamental perception of the physiology of the human body is so unlike the West's, it stands to reason that their method of diagnosis and prescription is also different. They tend to see remedies as grouped according to their effect, rather than linked to the cure of a particular disease or illness, and because they believe that illness is a sign of imbalance within the human body their prescriptions are designed to rectify that imbalance. For example, Chinese practitioners classify medicines as dispelling water or moist downward flow, strengthening earth or purging congealed damp. It is the effect with which they are concerned, rather than the specific complaint. The same medicine may be used for a variety of different illnesses if the treatments all require the same effect to be produced within the body. Conversely, the same illness in two patients may be treated with completely different remedies because the effect created is not the same — although the illness is the same, its source is not.

MEDIATING PRESCRIPTIONS

This type of prescription forms the most widely used group of remedies in traditional Chinese medicine. There are mild and moderately strong forms of mediating prescriptions, used to treat symptoms which are both internal and external such as disharmony of the liver and spleen. They have the unique property of being able to induce both warmth and cold, as well as to combat and preserve simultaneously, and to achieve a balance between the external and the internal. They are prescribed to achieve a balance between yin and yang and between all the internal organs.

Mediation of half-external and half-internal symptoms

These symptoms include fullness in the chest, fluctuating heat and cold, dry throat, dizziness, loss of appetite and a bitter taste in the mouth. As it is difficult to treat these symptoms with medicines which only cause sweating or ones which lower the flow, it is necessary to use a mediating treatment such as Bupleurum Tonic (see page 118).

Mediation of the liver and spleen

In cases of stagnation of qi in the spleen and liver, the following symptoms may be present: loss of appetite, bowel disorders, bloating of the waist and chest, disharmony between the spleen and liver and between the liver and stomach. For these symptoms a mediating prescription such as Chao Yan Powder (see page 119), Zi Yi Tonic (see page 121) and Pain and Diarrhoea Prescription (see page 120) should be used.

Mediation of the stomach and intestines

When there is an imbalance between heat and cold, or disorders of the stomach and intestines with symptoms such as pain in the abdomen caused by a concentration of cold in the intestines, a feeling of nausea without actual vomiting, and a concentration of heat in the stomach, then prescriptions such as Huang Lian Soup (see page 120) should be used.

Mediation and treatment of malaria

Malaria is one of those illnesses which is seen as both internal and external simultaneously. Symptoms include a feeling of nausea without actual vomiting, fullness at the waist and chest and fluctuations between heat and cold. Prescriptions would include Bupleurum Tonic (see page 118) and Seven Wonder Tonic (see page 121). It could well be necessary to add or subtract ingredients in both prescriptions for individual cases.

INTERNAL WARMTH OR COLD-DISPELLING PRESCRIPTIONS

Remedies in this category use herbs with warming or heating properties to remove and replace internal cold, to treat cold which has concentrated in the meridians and internal organs, and to remedy deficiency of yang in the body. Warmth prescriptions are divided into three groups:

- Those which warm the meridians and dispel cold from them
- Those which restore yang and correct mischannelling (or incorrect-flowing qi) in the meridians

- Those which warm the internal organs and help dispel cold from them

Internal warmth prescriptions are used to restore mental energy, to aid the circulation, to assist the digestive system and to correct any defective internal distribution of energy. They have a generally stimulating effect on the body and its functions, which helps to improve overall health. They are used in the treatment of ulcers, indigestion, dyspepsia, rheumatoid arthritis and chilblains.

Prescriptions include Chinese Angelica Zi Yi Tonic (see page 122) and Five Combination Tonic (see page 123). Five Combination Tonic is also useful in restoring qi and improving circulation.

Li Chung Pills (see page 123) would be prescribed when the symptoms include those already mentioned as well as a pale tongue, pains in the abdomen accompanied by coldness, and a slow, weak pulse. Li Chung Pills are usually prescribed to restore central qi. An adjustment may be made for individual cases, with other herbs such as aconite and cinnamon being added or left out. When bowel problems are added to the list of symptoms then Huang Lian (*Coptis chinensis*/golden thread) may be added to the prescriptions. Each time a herb is added or left out the combination has a separate name.

Evodia Tonic (see page 122) may be used in order to stop vomiting in patients suffering from all the symptoms mentioned above, and also in the treatment of heart disease, ulcers, liver disease and high blood pressure.

LOWER FLOWING OR DOWNWARD METHOD PRESCRIPTIONS

These prescriptions are laxative in their effect and help to dispel heat and dampness. They are divided into groups, depending on whether they are required to act quickly or slowly, on the symptoms treated and on the origins of those symptoms. Only those in the Moist Downward Flow category should be taken over a long period.

Cool Lower Flow

These prescriptions are used to treat people who are solid and hot internally. Symptoms are bloated abdomen, hard bowel motions, high temperature, pain, thirst, delirium, headache, vomiting of blood and stagnation of qi in the internal organs. The prescriptions include Da Zheng Qi Soup (see page 124) and Lian Gor Powder (see page 124).

Moist Downward Flow

These prescriptions are used to treat an over-abundance of whatever is affecting the fluid (dew) symptoms of dryness after illness or owing to old age. They are also used for symptoms of deficiency of the blood affecting the bowels after childbirth, and when there is long-standing hardness of bowel motions. Prescriptions include Wu Yan Pills (see page 126).

Warm Lower Flow

These are used to treat symptoms of weakness, emptiness and a gathering of cold in the spleen, often accompanied by hardness of the bowels, coldness in the limbs and a sinking, slow pulse. They are also used to treat concentrated yin cold, which reveals itself in expansion of the bowels, oedema or dropsy and difficulty in passing motions. Prescriptions include Warm Spleen Soup (see page 126) and Rhubarb and Aconite Soup (see page 125).

Cold Lower Flow

These prescriptions help to vitalize the large intestine. They are used as antibiotics, antiseptics, neutralizing agents and in the treatment of diarrhoea. They are also prescribed to control allergies in their active stage, and for lung infections. They are suitable for use with symptoms of high fever, constipation, thirst, delirium and a full or painful abdomen. They can be used in cases of nosebleeds, high blood pressure accompanied by headaches, or even for acute conjunctivitis. Increasingly they are being applied in cases of acute appendicitis, chronic constipation and liver disease.

Dispelling of Dampness

These prescriptions are used to treat fluids which collect in the body or mucus (tan) concentrated in the swollen abdomen or chest. They are also used to treat stagnation of qi in the internal organs. They include Ten Jujube Soup (see page 125).

SWEAT EVAPORATION PRESCRIPTIONS

As well as promoting sweating, these remedies cause expansion of the veins, improve the circulation of the blood and increase the amount of heat escaping from the body, which lowers temperature. They can be used to treat flu, and commonly for loss of voice, infected tonsils, lung infections including bronchitis, measles and mumps. They can also be used safely alongside Western medicines in the treatment of kidney problems, allergies and acute rheumatism. They are beneficial in increasing the effectiveness of Western treatments, and they speed up recovery after illness. The prescriptions in this category have various specific functions.

To encourage sweating

Sweating helps disperse certain cold-related symptoms such as stuffy or running nose, headache, high fever, white tongue, general pain all over the body and floating pulse. This category can be further divided into extension of warmth and extension of cold methods. The former are used to treat illnesses with cold-related symptoms, and include Ma Huang Soup (see page 128) and Cinnamon Soup (see page 127). The latter are used to treat illnesses with heat-related symptoms and include Honeysuckle and Forsythia Powder (see page 128) and Mulberry and Chrysanthemum Drink (see page 129).

To remove wetness through evaporation of sweat

Used to treat cold-winded and wetness-related diseases with symptoms such as heaviness of the body, white tongue, pain, floating slow pulse, swelling of the head and external appearance of wetness, these prescriptions include Ma Huang Soup (see page 128) and Cinnamon Soup (see page 127).

To assist the rapid maturing and disappearance of rashes in the early stages of chickenpox

Prescriptions used for this include Cimicifuga and Pueraria Soup (see page 127).

To relieve swelling

This is achieved through evaporation, which not only disperses wetness through sweating but also clears the lung passages of qi. These prescriptions cause the concentrated fluids to be moved to the bladder, promote the passing of wind and relieve swelling. They include Yer Pi Soup (see page 130) and the Prescription to Expel Wind and Promote the Passage of Water (see page 130), and are used to treat yang water illness, the symptoms of which are a swollen body with wind and a floating pulse.

MINOR COMPLAINTS AND INJURIES

For minor complaints such as rashes or insect bites the herbalist may prescribe a single herb in the form of an ointment or oil. Most herbal practitioners do not deal with injuries as such except to prescribe medicines to clear blood clotting and bruising. This method is also used for the treatment of broken bones, which are usually set with splints made from bamboo. A dressing of herbs is then applied externally.

PRESCRIPTION RECIPES

As we have stated elsewhere, please don't attempt to make up any of these recipes from herbal ingredients that you have picked yourself or have purchased anywhere but from a reliable source of Chinese medicinal products. Although throughout the text we have used common names, these are only intended as a general guide for the reader to understand the type of plant we are talking about: the correct Chinese version may well be significantly different, with completely different properties, and an alternative may be useless or even dangerous. In addition, only experienced Chinese herbalists know which part of the plant to use.

Don't be put off by these words of caution. In fact people exercise the same care with their everyday food in the West, but we think nothing of it because we are so used to doing so. We happily eat stewed rhubarb, which has a slight laxative effect; if we stewed the leaves and ate them, however, the laxative effect would be much stronger and we would die in great pain. Similarly we regularly buy and eat the popular tomato, but would not be tempted to eat the berries of its cousin the poisonous deadly nightshade. So for Chinese herbal remedies use the services of a reliable stockist or practitioner.

The commonest method of preparing Chinese herbal medicine is to make a tea (*t'ang*) or soup. Another option is to pulverize the herbs and moisten them with a substance such as honey to make them into pills. Or they can be finely powdered and added to water.

When preparing soups, the ingredients have to be simmered in a non-metallic (for instance, glazed clay) pot with the specified amount of water. When the liquid has reduced to the stated amount, the soup is ready to be cooled and drunk. Quantities of water are usually given in terms of rice bowls, which is the herbalist's standard measure (one rice bowl is about 10 fl oz or 300 ml.).

When the herbs have to be made into pills, stir-fried or powdered this is usually done by the herbalist. Under normal circumstances only the boiling of herbs to make soups is done at home. If the instruction is to stir fry the ingredients in honey, only a spoonful or two of honey is usually needed. The quantities given for each of the prescriptions below make one dose of medicine, unless otherwise stated.

Mediating prescriptions

Bupleurum Tonic

Symptoms: fluctuating coldness and heat, loss of appetite, bitter taste in the mouth, fullness in the chest, dizziness and dry throat.

Ingredients:
18 g Chai Hu (*Bupleurum chinense*/thorowax)
12 g Ban Zhi Lian (*Scutellaria baicalensis*/skullcap)

12 g *Campanumoea pilosula*
9 g Ban Xia (*Pinellia ternata*/'Half summer')
3 slices Gan Jiang (*Zingiber officinale*/fresh ginger)
3 Da Zao (Hong) (*Ziziphus jujuba*/Chinese jujubes)
6 g Gan Cao Zhi (*Glycyrrhiza uralensis*/liquorice)

Preparation: add the ingredients to 3 rice bowls of water and reduce by simmering until ¾ of a rice bowl of liquid is left.

Chao Yan Powder

Symptoms: loss of appetite, bowel disorders, loss of shen and bloating of waist and chest.

Ingredients:
9 g Chai Hu (*Bupleurum chinense*/thorowax)
9 g Bai Shao (*Paeonia lactiflora*/white peony root)
9 g Dang Gui (*Angelica sinensis*/Chinese angelica)
9 g Bai Zhu (*Atractylodes macrocephala*)
9 g Fu Ling (*Poria cocos*/hoelen)
6 g Gan Jiang (*Zingiber officinale*/fresh ginger)
6 g Gan Cao (*Glycyrrhiza uralensis*/liquorice)

Preparation: stir fry the liquorice in honey and add the rest of the ingredients and 3 rice bowls of water. Simmer and reduce until ¾ of a rice bowl of liquid remains. This will make one dose for one day (ie take all in one dose).

Huang Lian Soup

Symptoms: feeling of nausea without vomiting, abdominal pain, concentration of heat, diarrhoea with dizziness and weakness.

Ingredients:
15 g Gan Cao (*Glycyrrhiza uralensis*/liquorice)
6 g Huang Lian (*Coptis chinensis*/golden thread)
9 g Ban Xia (*Pinellia ternata*/'Half summer')
6 g Gan Jiang Zhi (*Zingiber officinale*/dried ginger)
6 g Gui Zhi (*Cinnamomum cassia*/cinnamon)
15 g *Campanumoea pilosula*
4 Da Zao (*Ziziphus jujuba*/Chinese jujubes)

Preparation: remove the stones from the jujubes and crush the fruit. Stir fry the liquorice in honey. Add the ingredients to 3 rice bowls of water and simmer and reduce until ¾ of a bowl of liquid remains.

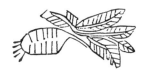

Pain and Diarrhoea Prescription

Symptoms: loss of appetite, bowel disorders, diarrhoea, painful abdomen, loss of shen.

Ingredients:
12 g Bai Zhu (*Atractylodes macrocephala*)
12 g Bai Shao/(*Paeonia lactiflora*/white peony root)
9 g Chen Pi (*Citrus reticulata*/tangerine peel)
6 g *Stenocoelium divaricatum root*

Preparation: add the ingredients to 3 rice bowls of water and simmer and reduce until ¾ of a rice bowl of liquid remains.

Seven Wonder Tonic

Symptoms: fluctuations of heat and cold, fullness at waist and chest, nausea. Also used for malaria.

Ingredients:
3 g Chang Shan (*Dichroa febrifuga*)
3 g Huo Po (*Magnolia officinalis*/magnolia)
3 g Qing Pi (*Citrus reticulata*/tangerine peel) (green)
3 g Chen Pi (*Citrus reticulata*/tangerine peel) (ripe)
3 g Gan Cao (*Glycyrrhiza uralensis*/liquorice)
9 g Da Fu Pi (*Areca catechu*/betel nut)
3 g Cao Guo (*Amomum tsao-ko*/'Grains fruit')

Preparation: add the ingredients to 3 rice bowls of water and simmer and reduce until only ¾ of a bowl of liquid remains.

Zi Yi Tonic

Symptoms: loss of appetite, bowel disorder, loss of shen and bloating of waist and chest. Used in the same circumstances as Chao Yan Powder (see page 119).

Ingredients:
15 g Fu Zi (*Aconitum carmichaeli*/Prepared root of Szechuan aconite)
12 g Gan Jiang Zhi (*Zingiber officinale*/dried ginger)
15 g Gan Cao Zhi (*Glycyrrhiza uralensis*/liquorice)

Preparation: stir fry the liquorice in honey. Add all the ingredients to 3–3½ rice bowls of water, and simmer and reduce until ¾ of a bowl of liquid remains.

Internal Warmth Prescriptions

Chinese Angelica Zi Yi Tonic

Symptoms: pain from stomach ulcers, chilblains, indigestion, rheumatoid arthritis.

Ingredients:
   9 g Dang Gui (*Angelica sinensis*/Chinese angelica)
   9 g Gui Zhi (*Cinnamomum cassia*/cinnamon)
   9 g Bai Shao (*Paeonia lactiflora*/white peony root)
   3 g Xi Xin (*Asarum sieboldii*/wild ginger)
   6 g Gan Cao (*Glycyrrhiza uralensis*/liquorice)
   9 g Da Zao (*Ziziphus jujuba*/Chinese jujube)
   6 g Wei Ling Xian (*Clematis armandii*/clematis root)

Preparation: add 4½ rice bowls of water to the ingredients, and simmer and reduce until 1 rice bowl of liquid remains.

Evodia Tonic

Symptoms: stomach ulcers, alleviating vomiting in those suffering from bowel problems and abdominal pain.

Ingredients:
   6 g Wu Zhu Yu (*Evodia rutaecarpa*/Evodia fruit)
   9 g Gan Jiang (*Zingiber officinale*/fresh ginger)
   15 g *Campanumoea pilosula*
   12 Da Zao (*Ziziphus jujuba*/Chinese jujube)

Preparation: remove the stones from the jujubes and crush the fruit. Add 3 rice bowls of water to the ingredients, and simmer and reduce until ¾ of a rice bowl of liquid remains.

Five Combination Tonic

Symptoms: poor circulation, pain from stomach ulcers, chilblains, indigestion, rheumatoid arthritis.

Ingredients:
9 g Huang Qi (*Astragulus membranaceus*/milk vetch)
9 g Gui Zhi (*Cinnamomum cassia*/cinnamon)
9 g Bai Shao (*Paeonia lactiflora*/white peony root)
18 g Gan Jiang (*Zingiber officinale*/fresh ginger)

Preparation: add 2½ rice bowls of water to the ingredients, and simmer and reduce until ¾ of a rice bowl of liquid remains.

Li Chung Pill

Symptoms: pains in abdomen, pale tongue, slow weak pulse, coldness.

Ingredients:
9 g Gan Jiang Zhi (*Zingiber officinale*/dried ginger)
12 g Cang Zhu (*Atractylodes lancea*)
15 g *Campanumoea pilosula*
6 g Gan Cao (*Glycyrrhiza uralensis*/liquorice)

Preparation: grind the ingredients into a powder and add honey to make a large pill, which should be chewed. Several smaller pills may be made if one pill is too large for the patient to manage, but they should all be taken at the same time.

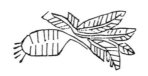

Lower Flowing Prescriptions

Da Zhang Qi Soup

Symptoms: high temperature, hard bowel motions, painful and bloated abdomen, headache, thirst, delirium, vomiting of blood.

Ingredients:
9 g Da Zhang (*Rheum officinale*/rhubarb)
12 g sodium sulphate
9 g Huo Po (*Magnolia officinalis*/magnolia)
9 g Zhi Shi (*Citrus aurantium*/Seville orange)

Preparation: add the ingredients to 3 rice bowls of water, and simmer and reduce until 1 rice bowl of liquid remains.

Lian Gor Powder

Symptoms: painful and bloated abdomen, high temperature, hard bowel motions, headache, vomiting blood, thirst, delirium.

Ingredients:
6 g Da Zhang (*Rheum officinale*/rhubarb)
9 g sodium sulphate
9 g Huang Qin (*Scutellaria baicalensis*/skullcap)
9 g Su Xin Hua (*Jasminum paniculatum*/jasmine)
18 g Lian Qiao (*Forsythia suspensa*/forsythia)
6 g Dan Zhu Ye (*Lophatherum gracile*/bamboo leaves)
6 g menthol
15 g honey
3 g Gan Cao (*Glycyrrhiza uralensis*/liquorice)

Preparation: grind the ingredients to a powder, add to warm water and take as a drink, or use less water and make into a capsule. These quantities give three to four doses to be taken during one day.

Rhubarb and Aconite Soup

Symptoms: coldness in the limbs, a sinking slow pulse, hardness of the bowels or an expansion of the bowels and constipation.

Ingredients:
9 g Da Zhang (*Rheum officinale*/rhubarb)
9 g Fu Zi (*Aconite carmichaeli*/prepared aconite)
6 g Xi Xin (*Asarum sieboldii*/wild ginger)

Preparation: add the ingredients to 3 rice bowls of water, and simmer and reduce until ¾ of a rice bowl of liquid remains.

Ten Jujube Soup

Symptoms: swollen abdomen, yellow tongue, concentration of mucus in the chest or congregating of dampness in the body.

Ingredients:
10 Da Zao (*Ziziphus jujuba*/Chinese jujubes)
0.5 g Gan Sui (*Euphorbia kansu*)
0.5 g Da Ji (*Euphorbia pekinensis*/Peking spurge root)
0.5 g Yuan Hua (*Daphne genkwa*/Daphne flower)
Preparation: remove the stones from the jujubes and crush the fruit. Add all the ingredients to 4½–5 rice bowls of water, and simmer and reduce until 1–1½ rice bowls of liquid remain. This medicine acts very swiftly.

125

Warm Spleen Soup

Symptoms: coldness in the limbs, sinking slow pulse caused by coldness in the spleen, hardness of the bowels. Expansion of the bowels and constipation caused by concentrated yin cold.

Ingredients:

9 g Fu Zi (*Aconite carmichaeli*/prepared aconite)
6 g Gan Jiang Zhi (*Zingiber officinale*/dried ginger)
9 g *Campanumoea pilosula*
3 g Gan Cao (*Glycyrrhiza uralensis*/liquorice)
9 g Da Zhang (*Rheum officinale*/rhubarb)

Preparation: add 3 rice bowls of water to the ingredients, and simmer and reduce until ¾ of a rice bowl of liquid remains.

Wu Yan Pills

Symptoms: dryness in old age or after illness. Persistent hardness of bowel movements. Weakness in the blood affecting bowel movements after childbirth.

Ingredients:

9 g Yu Li Ren (*Prunus consociiflora*/wild cherry bark)
9 g Hu Po (*Pinus armandii*/pine kernels)
9 g Ce Bai Ye (*Biota orientalis*/leafy twig of Arborvitae)
12 g Xing Ren (*Prunus armeniaca*/apricot kernels)
9 g Tao Ren (*Prunus persica*/peach kernels)
9 g Chen Pi (*Citrus reticulata*/tangerine peel)

Preparation: grind the ingredients to a powder and mix with honey. Make into a large pill, or several smaller ones, and chew rather than swallow whole.

Sweat Evaporation Prescriptions

Cimicifuga and Pueraria Soup

Symptoms: used for children and adults suffering from chickenpox or measles, if the rash associated with the disease is slow to appear.

Ingredients:
6 g Sheng Ma (*Cimicifuga dahurica*)
15 g Ge Gen (*Pueraria lobata*/kudzu root)
9 g Bai Shao (*Paeonia lactiflora*/white peony root)
9 g Gan Cao (*Glycyrrhiza uralensis*/liquorice)

Preparation: add the ingredients to 3 rice bowls of water, and simmer and reduce until ¾ of a rice bowl of liquid remains. This gives one dose, which should be taken each day for three days.

Cinnamon Soup 1

Symptoms: high fever, headache, stuffy or running nose, aches all over the body, floating pulse and white tongue – all associated with coldness.

Ingredients:
9 g Gui Zhi (*Cinnamomum cassia*/cinnamon)
9 g Bai Shao (*Paeonia lactiflora*/white peony root)
2 slices Gan Jiang (*Zingiber officinale*/fresh ginger)
4 Da Zao (*Ziziphus jujuba*/Chinese jujubes)
6 g Gan Cao (*Glycyrrhiza uralensis*/liquorice)

Preparation: remove the stones from the jujubes and crush the fruit. Add 3 rice bowls of water to the ingredients, and simmer and reduce until ¾ of a rice bowl of liquid remains.

Honeysuckle and Forsythia Powder

Symptoms: running or stuffy nose, high fever, pain all over the body, headache, white tongue and floating pulse – all associated with heat.

Ingredients:

9 g Jin Yin Hua (*Lonicera japonica*/honeysuckle)
9 g Lian Qiao (*Forsythia suspensa*/forsythia)
6 g Niu Bang Zi (*Arctium lappa*/great burdock)
6 g Jie Geng (*Platycodon grandiflorum*/balloon flower)
5 g Bo He (*Mentha arvensis*/mint)
6 g Dan Dou Chi (*Glycine max*/soyabean)
6 g Gan Cao (*Glycyrrhiza uralensis*/liquorice)
6 g Dan Zhu Ye (*Lophatherum gracile*/bamboo leaves)
6 g Jing Jie (*Schizonepeta tenuifolia*)

Preparation: grind the ingredients to a fine powder, add to warm water and drink. This will be enough for three doses, which should be taken over one day.

Ma Huang Soup

Symptoms: stuffy or running nose, headache, general achiness, high fever, white tongue, floating pulse. This medicine is used to treat these symptoms when caused by coldness.

Ingredients:

6 g Gan Cao (*Glycyrrhiza uralensis*/liquorice)
9 g Ma Huang (*Ephedra sinica*/ephedra)
9 g Gui Zhi (*Cinnamomum cassia*/cinnamon)
9 g Xing Ren (*Prunus armeniaca*/apricot kernels)

Preparation: stir fry the liquorice in honey, then add it to the other ingredients and 3 rice bowls of water. Simmer and reduce until ¾ of a rice bowl of liquid remains.

Ma Huang and Cinnamon Soup

Symptoms: heaviness of the body, pain, white tongue, swelling of the head, slow and floating pulse and moist appearance — all caused by cold-winded and wetness-related illnesses.

Ingredients:
6 g Gan Cao (*Glycyrrhiza uralensis*/liquorice)
9 g Gui Zhi (*Cinnamomum cassia*/cinnamon)
9 g Ma Huang (*Ephedra sinica*/ephedra)
9 g Xing Ren (*Prunus armeniaca*/apricot kernels)
9 g Cang Zhu (*Atractylodes chinensis*)

Preparation: stir fry the liquorice in honey, and then add with the rest of the ingredients to 3 rice bowls of water. Simmer and reduce until ¾ of a rice bowl of water remains. One dose should be taken each day after the evening meal.

Mulberry and Chrysanthemum Drink

Symptoms: running or stuffy nose, headache, high fever, pain all over the body, white tongue and floating pulse — all associated with heat.

Ingredients:
9 g Sang Ye (*Morus alba*/mulberry leaves)
6 g Ye Ju Hua (*Chrysanthemum indicum*/chrysanthemum)
6 g Bo He (*Mentha arvensis*/mint)
18 g Lian Qiao (*Forsythia suspensa*/forsythia)
9 g Jie Geng (*Platycodon grandiflorum*/balloon flower)
9 g Xing Ren (*Prunus armeniaca*/apricot kernels)
18 g Lu Gen (*Phragmites communis*/common reed)
3 g Gan Cao (*Glycyrrhiza uralensis*/liquorice)

Preparation: add the ingredients to 3 rice bowls of water, and simmer and reduce until ¾ of a rice bowl of liquid remains. This gives one dose, but the herbs can be boiled up a second time to give a second dose.

Prescription to Expel Wind and Promote the Passage of Water

Symptoms: swollen body with wind and floating pulse in women and the elderly.

Ingredients:
12 g Che Qian (*Plantago paludosa*/plantain)
9 g Fu Ping (*Spirodela polyrrhiza*/Duckweed)
18 g Lian Qiao (*Forsythia suspensa*/forsythia)
9 g Zi Su Ye (*Perilla frutescens*)
12 g Sang Zhi (*Morus alba*/mulberry root cortex)
30 g Bai Mao Gen (*Imperata cylindrica*/Woolly grass rhizome)
30 g Chong Wei Zi (*Leonurus sibiricus*/Siberian motherwort seeds)
18 g Jin Yin Hua (*Lonicera japonica*/honeysuckle)
6 g Gan Cao (*Glycyrrhiza uralensis*/liquorice)

Preparation: add 4½ rice bowls of water to the ingredients, and simmer and reduce until only 1 bowl of liquid remains.

Yer Pi Soup

Symptoms: wind with a swollen body and a floating pulse as a result of yang water illnesses.

Ingredients:
9 g Ma Huang (*Ephedra sinica*/ephedra)
6 g Gan Cao (*Glycyrrhiza uralensis*/liquorice)
15 g Shi Gao (hydrated calcium sulphate/gypsum)
3 slices Gan Jiang (*Zingiber officinale*/fresh ginger)
3 Da Zao (*Ziziphus jujuba*/Chinese jujubes)

Preparation: (method 1) remove the stones from the jujubes and crush the fruit. Add 3 rice bowls of water to the ingredients, simmer and reduce down to ¾ of a rice bowl of liquid: this provides one dose; (method 2) again, stone and crush the jujubes and crush the herbs to a powder with 6–9 g Cang Zhu (*Atractylodes chinensis*) to make Yer Pi Powder. The powder is added to a cup of warm water and provides two to three doses.

General herbal prescriptions

These are herbal prescriptions for common ailments such as colds, flu, coughs, sore throats and sore eyes.

Anemarrhena and Coltsfoot

Symptoms: coughs in the elderly with an excess of phlegm, shortness of breath and slight asthmatic symptoms.

Ingredients:
10 g Zhi Mu (*Anemarrhena asphodeloides*/Anemarrhena root)
10 g Kuan Dong Hua (*Tussilago farfara*/coltsfoot)
6 g Bei Mu (*Fritillaria verticillata*/fritillary bulb)
5 Da Zao (*Zizyphus jujuba*/Chinese jujubes)
3 slices Gan Jiang (*Zingiber officinale*/fresh ginger)

Preparation: remove the stones from the jujubes and crush the fruit. Stir fry the first two ingredients in honey, then add them to all the others in 3 rice bowls of water. Simmer and reduce until ¾ of a rice bowl of liquid remains. This makes two doses, which is one day's treatment. Alternatively, all the ingredients can be crushed together into a powder, which can then be added to water and taken twice a day in 6 g doses.

Angelica and Peony Soup

Symptoms: bruises and blood clots. Discomfort during pregnancy. Enduring pain in the abdomen which doesn't respond to other herbal treatments. Hardening of the arteries. Kidney problems in men. Depression. This prescription lowers cholesterol, restores blood and treats the liver.

Ingredients:
3 g Dang Gui (*Angelica sinensis*/Chinese angelica)
5 g Bai Shao (*Paeonia lactiflora*/white peony root)
2 g Gao Ben (*Ligusticum sinense*/Chinese lovage root)
3 g Bai Zhu (*Atractylodes macrocephala*)
3 g Fu Ling (*Poria cocos*/hoelen)
5 g Ze Xie (*Alisma plantago-aquatica*/water plantain)

Preparation: (method 1) add 3 rice bowls of water to the ingredients, simmer and reduce down to ¾ of a rice bowl of liquid, which provides one dose; (method 2) crush the herbs to a powder and add to warm water, which provides two to three doses.

Apricot Kernel and White Carrot Powder

Symptoms: coughs and tightness in the chest, shortness of breath and difficulty in getting rid of phlegm. This prescription is not effective for persistent coughs, but it is easily made and will often cure a mild cough at an early stage.

Ingredients:
10 Xing Ren (*Prunus armeniaca*/apricot kernels)
10 slices *Daucus alba*/white carrot

Preparation: crush the ingredients together and divide into two equal portions. Twice a day add one of the portions to a cup of Hong Tang water (brown-sugared water) and drink.

Chrysanthemum and Peppermint

Symptoms: red, painful eyes which are watering and affecting vision.

Ingredients:
10 g Ye Ju Hua (*Chrysanthemum indicum*/wild chrysanthemum)
3 g Bo He (*Mentha piperita*/peppermint)
6 g Bai Ji Li (*Tribulus terrestris*/caltrop fruit)

Preparation: use the freshest herbs possible. Add all the ingredients to 3 rice bowls of water, and simmer and reduce until ¾ of a rice bowl of liquid remains. Drink. The concoction can also be used warm to bathe the eyes.

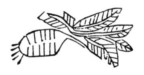

Cinnamon Soup 2

Symptoms: arthritic swelling and pain.

Ingredients:
9 g Gui Zhi (*Cinnamomum cassia*/cinnamon)
9 g Fu Zi (*Aconite carmichaeli*/prepared aconite)
6 g Gan Cao (*Glycyrrhiza uralensis*/liquorice)
9 g Gan Jiang (*Zingiber officinale*/fresh ginger)
3 Da Zao (*Ziziphus jujuba*/Chinese jujubes)

Preparation: remove the stones from the jujubes and crush the fruit. Add 3 rice bowls of water to the ingredients, and simmer and reduce until ¾ of a bowl of liquid remains.

Cinnamon and Peony Soup

Symptoms: chilblains. This soup is both preventative and curative, and works by keeping the body warm. It should be taken for five consecutive days, or ten if the chilblains start to burst.

Ingredients:
2 g Gan Cao (*Glycyrrhiza uralensis*/liquorice)
3 g Gui Zhi (*Cinnamomum cassia*/cinnamon)
3 g Bai Shao (*Paeonia lactiflora*/white peony root)
2 g Dang Gui (*Angelica sinensis*/Chinese angelica)
4 Da Zao (*Ziziphus jujuba*/Chinese jujubes)

Preparation: remove the stones from the jujubes and crush the fruit. Stir fry the liquorice in honey, and then add with the rest of the ingredients to 3 rice bowls of water. Simmer and reduce until ¾ of a rice bowl of water remains.

Cold Remedy

Symptoms: colds with high fever, aching body and headache. This is probably one of the oldest Chinese prescriptions in existence.

Ingredients:
9 g Zi Su Geng (*Perilla acuta*/Perilla fruit)
9 g *Stenocoelium divaricatum*
9 g Jing Jie (*Schizonepeta tenuifolia*)
6 g Bo He (*Mentha piperita*/peppermint)

Preparation: add all the ingredients to 3 rice bowls of water. Simmer and reduce until ¾ of a rice bowl of water remains. In winter and spring add Hong Tang (brown sugar) and fresh ginger for taste. In summer and autumn add bamboo leaves and white sugar for taste.

Eight Precious Soup

Symptoms: dizziness, depression, pale face, impaired vision, loss of appetite, reluctance to speak, pale tongue with yellowish fur, weak pulse that is difficult to find. Given to women after childbirth, as a tonic and for nervous exhaustion as a result of stress. This prescription is a combination of Four natural Products Tonic and Four Gentlemen's Tonic.

Ingredients:
15 g Campanumoea pilosula
12 g Cang Zhu (*Atractylodes chinensis*)
9 g Fu Ling (*Poria cocos*/hoelen)
6 g Gan Cao (*Glycyrrhiza uralensis*/liquorice)
12 g Sheng Di Huang (*Rehmania glutinosa*/Chinese foxglove)
9 g Dang Gui (*Angelica sinensis*/Chinese angelica)
12 g Bai Shao (*Paeonia lactiflora*/white peony root)
6 g Gao Ben (*Ligusticum acutilobum*/Chinese lovage root)

Preparation: add 6 rice bowls of water to the ingredients, and simmer and reduce until 1½ rice bowls of liquid remain.

Flu and Colds

Ingredients:
6–12 g Sang Ye (*Morus alba*/mulberry leaves)
3–10 g Man Jing Zi (*Vitex rotundifolia*/muscadine grape)
15–30 g Che Qian (*Plantago paludosa*/plantain, whole herb)
3–10 g Che Qian (*Plantago paludosa*/plantain, seeds)

Preparation: add ingredients to 3 rice bowls of water, simmer and reduce down to 1 bowl.

Four Gentlemen's Tonic

Symptoms: weakness for no apparent reason, especially in very good weather. This prescription restores qi in the blood.

Ingredients:
15 g *Campanumoea pilosula*
12 g Cang Zhu (*Atractylodes chinensis*)
9 g Fu Ling (*Poria cocos*/hoelen)
6 g Gan Cao (*Glycyrrhiza uralensis*/liquorice)

Preparation: add 3 rice bowls of water to the ingredients, and simmer and reduce until ¾ of a rice bowl of liquid remains.

Four Natural Products Tonic

Symptoms: Threatened miscarriage. Menstrual disorders. Excessive kicking of foetus. Anaemia, poor circulation, loss of tone in the muscles of the womb, especially after childbirth. Blood-related symptoms, deficient blood.

Ingredients:
12 g Sheng Di Huang (*Rehmania glutinosa*/Root of Chinese foxglove)
9 g Dang Gui (*Angelica sinensis*/Chinese angelica)
12 g Bai Shao (*Paeonia lactiflora*/white peony root)
6 g Gao Ben (*Ligusticum acutilobum*/Chinese lovage root)

Preparation: add 3 rice bowls of water to the ingredients, and simmer and reduce until ¾ of a rice bowl of liquid remains.

Ginger and Spring Onion Soup

Symptoms: colds with headache and high temperature. Coughs, phlegm and a running nose, especially in winter. This is a very popular home remedy in China.

Ingredients:
10 g Gan Jiang (*Zingiber officinale*/fresh ginger)
1 whole large Xie Bai (*Allium macrostemon*/bulb of Chinese chive)
3 g Hua Jiao (*Zanthoxylum piperitum*/Japanese prickly ash)
30 g outer skin *Daucus alba*/white carrot

Preparation: boil all the ingredients for 20–30 minutes in 1 rice bowl of water. To promote sweating, the soup should be drunk while still quite hot.

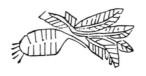

Ginger and White Carrot Soup

Symptoms: chronic bronchitis with tightness in the chest and dry bowel motions. This prescription will relieve a lot of the discomfort, although it will not effect a complete cure.

Ingredients:
15 g Gan Jiang (*Zingiber officinale*/fresh ginger)
6 slices *Daucus alba*/white carrot
30 g honey

Preparation: add all the ingredients to 3 rice bowls of water. Simmer and reduce until ¾ of a rice bowl of water remains. Take the whole mixture once a day for 5–7 days.

Ginseng and Aconite Soup

Symptoms: cold hands and feet, cold, heavy sweating with tasteless sweat and very weak pulse. This is a very expensive prescription which helps to restore yang, gives strength to the heart and raises the blood pressure. It is used especially for those over the age of fifty who have a tendency to faint. It can also help reduce hardening of the arteries.

Ingredients:
12 g Ren Shen (*Panax ginseng*/ginseng)
9 g Fu Zi (*Aconite carmichaeli*/prepared aconite)

Preparation: add the ingredients to 3 rice bowls of water, and simmer and reduce until ¾ of a rice bowl of liquid remains.

Increase of Dew Soup

Symptoms: high fever, extreme thirst, very dry tongue, very hard red bowel motions, constipation, slow pulse. These symptoms usually occur in the summer, and this very powerful medicine is used mainly for yang and heat diseases. It provides dew, dispels heat and moistens the intestines.

Ingredients:
10 g Xuan Shen (*Scrophularia nodosa*/figwort)
8 g Mai Men Dong (*Ophiopogon japonicus*/'Lush winter wheat')
8 g Sheng Di Huang (*Rehmania glutinosa*/Root of Chinese foxglove)

Preparation: add 3 rice bowls of water to the ingredients and simmer and reduce until ¾ of a rice bowl of liquid remains.

Jian Chi Soup

Symptoms: cold cough, cold phlegm, cough which causes difficulty with breathing during the night.

Ingredients:
9 g Ban Xia (fa) (*Pinellia ternata*/'Half summer')
3 g Gan Cao (*Glycyrrhiza uralensis*/liquorice)
6 g Bai Zhi (*Angelica dahurica*/angelica root)
3 g Chen Pi (*Citrus reticulata*/tangerine peel)
6 g Huo Po (*Magnolia officinalis*/magnolia)
9 g Zi Su Ye (*Perilla frutescens*/Perilla leaf)
9 g Dang Gui (*Angelica sinensis*/Chinese angelica)
1.5 g Gui Zhi (*Cinnamomum cassia*/cinnamon)
9 g Gan Jiang (*Zingiber officinale*/fresh ginger)

Preparation: boil all the ingredients except the cinnamon in 3 rice bowls of water until ¾ of a rice bowl remains. Crush the cinnamon into a powder and place in a bowl. Pour the boiled preparation over the cinnamon.

Ling Kwei Zhu Chin Soup

Symptoms: simple coughs in their early stages.

Ingredients:
9 g Gan Cao (*Glycyrrhiza uralensis*/liquorice)
18 g Fu Ling (*Poria cocos*/hoelen)
12 g Cang Zhu (*Atractylodes chinensis*)
9 g Gui Zhi (*Cinnamomum cassia*/cinnamon)

Preparation: add 3 rice bowls of water to the ingredients, and simmer and reduce until ¾ of a bowl of liquid remains.

Ma Huang and Apricot Kernel Soup

Symptoms: flu in winter and spring with a cough and high fever, shortness of breath and phlegm. This prescription depresses coughs and dispels phlegm.

Ingredients:
6 g Ma Huang (*Ephedra sinica*/ephedra)
10 g Xing Ren (*Prunus armeniaca*/apricot kernels)
3 g *Thea bohea*/red tea
6 g Zi Su Ye (*Perilla frutescens*/Perilla leaf)
3 g Gan Cao (*Glycyrrhiza uralensis*/liquorice)
3 slices Gan Jiang (*Zingiber officinale*/fresh ginger)

Preparation: add the ingredients to 3 rice bowls of water, and simmer and reduce until only ¾ of a rice bowl of liquid remains. Take after a meal.

Peony and Liquorice Soup

Symptoms: kidney pain. Tiredness and exhaustion in women. Pains in the hips of women.

Ingredients:
10 g Bai Shao (*Paeonia lactiflora*/white peony root)
10 g Gan Cao (*Glycyrrhiza uralensis*/liquorice)
2 g Yan Hu Suo (*Corydalis turtschaninovii*/corydalis root)

Preparation: add 3 rice bowls of water to the ingredients, and simmer and reduce until ¾ of a rice bowl of liquid remains. This makes two doses.

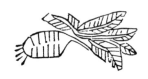

Plantain and Honeysuckle Soup

Symptoms: summer and autumn diarrhoea.

Ingredients:
30 g Che Qian (*Plantago paludosa, P. sibirica, P. depressa/* plantain)
30 g Jin Yin Hua (*Lonicera japonica/*honeysuckle)

Preparation: add the ingredients with brown and white sugar to 3 rice bowls of water, and simmer and reduce until only ¾ of a rice bowl of liquid remains. This is enough for two doses to be taken during the course of one day.

Plum and Sweet Pear

Symptoms: chronic bronchitis with shortness of breath and rapid breathing with persistent phlegm.

Ingredients:
3 plums
1 sweet pear

Preparation: stone the plums and roast them over a flame until the skin is burnt, then peel it off and throw it away. Crush the body of the fruit and place it in the sliced open pear. Steam it all and eat one per night.

Pregnancy Test

Symptoms: to be used as a test for pregnancy when a period is overdue and there is no accompanying discomfort. If the patient is pregnant, the prescription will have no ill effects. If she is not, it will cause the period to start.

Ingredients:
9 g Bai Zhi (*Angelica dahuria*/angelica)
6 g Huang Qin (*Scutellaria baicalensis*/skullcap)
9 g Chuan Xiong (*Ligustrum wallichii*/Szechuan lovage root)
6 g Gan Cao (*Glycyrrhiza uralensis*/liquorice)
6 g Jing Jie (*Schizonepeta tenuifolia*)
10 g Bai Zhu (*Atractylodes macrocephala*)
6 g Zi Su Ye (*Perilla frutescens*/Perilla leaf)
10 g Dang Gui (*Angelica sinensis*/Chinese angelica)

Preparation: add all the ingredients to 3 rice bowls of water, and simmer and reduce until ¾ of a rice bowl of liquid remains. Reboil the herbs three times a day.

Roast Garlic

Symptoms: diarrhoea with abdominal pains which have persisted for three to five days.

Ingredients:
1 large Xie Bai (*Allium sativum*/bulb of garlic)

Preparation: roast the unpeeled garlic bulb over a flame. Peel and eat one per day.

Rubia and Brown Sugar

Symptoms: for women who are not pregnant and whose period is two to three months overdue, especially if accompanied by pain with fever and coldness. This prescription should not be continued once the period has started.

Ingredients:
30 g Qian Cao Gen (*Rubia cordifolia*/Madder root)
30 g Hong Tang (brown sugar)

Preparation: add the rubia to 3 rice bowls of water, then simmer and reduce to ¾ of a rice bowl of liquid. Add the sugar and take while still warm once a day for three to five days.

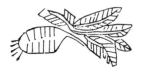

San Hou Soup

Symptoms: cough, slight shortness of breath (but not asthma), stuffy lung passages, coughing due to flu, whooping cough.

Ingredients:
6 g Ma Huang (*Ephedra sinica*/ephedra)
9 g Xing Ren (*Prunus armeniaca*/apricot kernels)
3 g Gan Cao (*Glycyrrhiza uralensis*/liquorice)

Preparation: add 3 rice bowls of water to the ingredients, and simmer and reduce until ¾ of a rice bowl of liquid remains.

San Sheng Yin

Symptoms: an excess of sputum. This prescription is also commonly used in the treatment of paralysis. Recently it has been used to relieve unbearable pain such as that caused by cancer. It has a powerful painkilling effect, but when it is not being used for this purpose it should be boiled for a much longer time in order to limit the powerfulness of the three main herbs.

Ingredients:
9 g Ren Shen (*Panax ginseng*/ginseng)
24 g Gan Jiang Zhi (*Zingiber officinale*/dried ginger)
4 g Tian Nan Xing (*Arisaema thunbergii*/'Jock-in-the-pulpit')
3 g *Aconiteum fischerii* (aconite)
4 g Fu Zi (*Aconite carmichaeli*/prepared aconite)
3 g Mu Xiong (*Saussurea lappa*/costus root)

Preparation: boil all the ingredients except the *Saussurea lappa* in 3–4 rice bowls of water for 1–2 hours, until the liquid is reduced to 1 rice bowl. Add the *Saussurea lappa* a few minutes before the end of boiling.

Soup to Mend Yang and Restore the Elements

Symptoms: partial paralysis after a stroke, with facial disorder, lack of control over speech, saliva, bowels and bladder. The last five ingredients help to move the blood and to dispel blood clots.

Ingredients:
30–60 g Huang Qi (*Astragulus membranaceus*/milk vetch)
6 g Dang Gui (*Angelica sinensis*/Chinese angelica)
9 g Bai Shao/Chi Shao (*Paeonia lactiflora*/peony, unpeeled)
6 g Chuan Xiong (*Ligustrum wallichii*/Szechuan lovage root)
9 g Tao Ren (*Prunus persica*/peach kernels)
4.5 g Hong Hua (*Carthamus tinctorius*/safflower)

Preparation: add the ingredients to 5–6 rice bowls of water, and simmer and reduce until 1½ rice bowls of liquid remains.

Stenocoelium and Schizonepeta Soup

Symptoms: spasmodic toothache.

Ingredients:
6 g *Stenocoelium divaricatum* root
6 g Jing Jie (*Schizonepeta tenuifolia*)
6 g Ju Hua (*Chrysanthemum morifolium*/chrysanthemum)
6 g Jie Geng (*Platycodon grandiflorum*/balloon flower)
6 g Chuan Xiong (*Ligustrum wallichii*/Szechuan lovage root)
6 g Fu Zi (*Aconite carmichaeli*/prepared root of Szechuan aconite)
6 g (*Aconitum kusnezoffii*/aconite)
10 g Xuan Shen (*Scrophularia nodosa*/figwort)
3 g Gan Cao (*Glycyrrhiza uralensis*/liquorice)

Preparation: add all the ingredients to 3 rice bowls of water, and simmer and reduce until ¾ of a rice bowl of liquid remains. Take for three days.

Three Seeds Cough-Smothering Soup

Symptoms: difficulty in breathing, coughs, phlegm, stuffy chest. This prescription restores the correct flow of ch'i in the meridians. It is mainly used for the elderly, and in the treatment of bronchitis.

Ingredients:
9 g Zi Su Ye (*Perilla frutescens*/Perilla seeds)
9 g Bai Jie Zi (*Sinapis alba*/mustard seeds)
9 g Lai Fu Zi (*Raphannus sativus*/radish seeds)

Preparation: add 3 rice bowls of water to the ingredients, and simmer and reduce until ¾ of a rice bowl of liquid remains.

Zhi Sou San

Symptoms: irritating cough at night. Cough caused by flu. This prescription expands the lungs and dispels phlegm.

Ingredients:
4 g Jing Jie (*Schizonepeta tenuifolia*)
3 g Chen Pi (*Citrus reticulata*/tangerine peel)
9 g Bai Bu (*Stemona sessilifolia*/stemona root)
9 g Bai Gian (*Cynanchum stauntoni*)
9 g Zi Wan (*Aster amellus*/Purple aster root)
9 g Jie Geng (*Platycodon grandiflorum*/balloon flower)
3 g Gan Cao (*Glycyrrhiza uralensis*/liquorice)

Preparation: grind the herbs into a powder, add to water and drink. The herbs can alternatively be boiled with 3–4 rice bowls of water until reduced to ¾ of a bowl of liquid, which should be drunk while still warm.

MEDICINAL FOODS

The Chinese have for centuries believed that prevention is better than cure, and these special recipes might be regarded as the Oriental equivalent of 'an apple a day...'. They are also used at the onset of mild symptoms to stop them developing into something more serious. Recipes and ingredients vary from family to family, as do quantities and cooking times. Please feel free to vary the recipes given here to suit your own requirements. The ingredients can mostly be bought from your local supermarket.

Boiled Eggs with Sang Ji Sheng

Sang Ji Sheng (*Loranthus parasiticus*/Mulberry parasite) is used to treat liver and kidney complaints and to strengthen tendons. It helps to preserve blood and dispel wind, to prevent threatened miscarriage and to promote the flow of breast milk. Often used to treat rheumatism, back pain and loss of sensation in the limbs, it is also recommended for the treatment of diabetes and high blood pressure caused by arteriosclerosis. In pregnant women, it is helpful in relieving back pain. When used on its own as a tea, it is a useful preventative medicine. It also nourishes skin, hair and muscles and strengthens the teeth.

Ingredients:
Eggs
15–30 g Sang Ji Sheng (*Loranthus parasiticus*)

Preparation: hard boil the eggs in water containing the Sang Ji Sheng. Eat the eggs and drink the water.

Chicken with Ye Jiao Teng

This recipe nourishes the blood and helps strengthen the kidneys. It is used to treat problems of the uterus and haemorrhoids. It also strengthens and improves hair quality.

Ingredients:
30 g Ye Jiao Teng (*Polygonum multiflorum*/'The vine of Solomon's seed')
1 medium-size chicken
ginger, salt, oil and wine for flavouring

Preparation: grind the Ye Jiao Teng to a powder and wrap it in white muslin. Remove the giblets from the chicken and stuff it with the ground herb in its muslin bag. Boil the chicken in water until the meat falls off the bone. Remove the Ye Jiao Teng-filled muslin bag. Shred the meat into the broth and add ginger, salt, oil and wine to taste.

Chinese Angelica with Lamb

Dang Gui (*Angelica sinensis*/Chinese angelica) is regarded as the foremost herb for the treatment of gynaecological problems. Its value in treating complaints, especially those related to pre-menstrual syndrome, was written about as long as two thousand years ago in a medical treatise called *Shen-nung Pen Ts'ao Chingar*.

Lamb, as well as its use in flavouring a dish, has its own medicinal qualities. It is said to give warmth to the spleen and stomach and to restore ch'i and blood, providing health and strength to the body.

Ingredients:
9–15 g Dang Gui (*Angelica sinensis*/Chinese angelica)
500 g lamb (boned and diced)
slices of Gan Jiang (*Zingiber officinale*/fresh ginger) to taste

Preparation: steam all the ingredients together in a cooking pot until the lamb is tender.

Chinese Chives and Ginger with Milk

This recipe is used to treat an upset stomach and vomiting immediately after eating. Chives taste hot and provide warmth; they are associated with the liver, stomach and kidney meridians, and activate qi. Ginger also tastes hot and provides warmth; it is associated with the lung, stomach and spleen meridians. It dispels cold, stops vomiting and disperses sputum. Milk has a sweet taste and is associated with the lung and stomach meridians.

Ingredients:
2 soupspoons of juice from fresh chives (use chives from supermarket)
1 teaspoon Gan Jiang (*Zingiber officinale*/fresh ginger juice)
250 ml fresh milk

Preparation: steam together in a cooking pot and take before a meal.

Chinese Yam and Chinese Wolfberry Soup

Yam has the power to strengthen the spleen and stomach, the lungs and kidneys. It contains large quantities of protein and carbohydrate. Wolfberry seeds help restore the liver and kidneys and are also used to treat diabetes.

Ingredients:
any lean meat (see Preparation)
18–30 g Bi Xie Xu Duan (*Dioscorea batatas*/Chinese yam)
6–15 g Di Gu Pi (*Lycium chinensis*/Chinese wolfberry)

Preparation: make a meat soup and then add the other ingredients to it.

Pig's Kidneys and Du Zhong

Du Zhong protects the liver and kidneys, strengthens bones and tendons, and is used as a remedy for back pain. It is very effective in the treatment of high blood pressure and cholesterol levels. It is also helpful in preventing threatened miscarriage in the middle stages of pregnancy. It is better fried than raw, but even better boiled.

Ingredients:
1 pig's kidney (cleaned and sliced)
9–15 g Du Zhong (*Eucommia ulmoides*/Eucommia bark)

Preparation: steam the ingredients together in a cooking pot until the kidney is cooked.

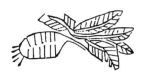

Pork, Lotus Seed and Lily Soup

Lily is used to treat dry coughs and lungs. It restores central ch'i, strengthens the kidneys, dispels heat and cures coughs. It is also used to treat problems of the heart and lungs, stomach and spleen, and as a tonic in the treatment of tuberculosis and neurasthenia. Lotus seeds strengthen the stomach and spleen and promote mental stability and healthy functioning of the kidneys. They are also useful in the treatment of excessive menstrual bleeding and leucorrhoea in women and wet dreams and seminal emission in men. Both lily and lotus seeds contain large amounts of protein and vitamin C.

Ingredients:
lean pork (see Preparation)
15–25 g Lian Zi (*Nelumb nucifera*/lotus seeds)
15–30 g Bai He (*Lilium brownii*/lily)

Preparation: make a soup with the meat and add the herbal ingredients to it.

Watercress and Date Soup

This recipe is used to treat a dry cough, dry throat and constipation. Watercress, as well as containing an abundance of vitamins A, C and D, has the ability to clear and moisten the lungs. Dates are sweet and provide dew.

Ingredients:
500 g watercress (chopped)
5–6 fresh dates (chopped)

Preparation: add 3 cups of water and boil for 2 hours or longer.

7

Over-the-Counter (Patent) Remedies

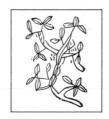

Caution: anyone with persistent or serious symptoms should consult their doctor or a qualified practitioner of Chinese herbal medicine. Self-diagnosis and self-treatment are not recommended or advised except in the most minor of conditions.

Apart from the infinite number of prescriptions of different combinations which herbalists can make up, they will also stock a variety of pre-packaged, bought-in herbal prescriptions. They may have been prepared in Hong Kong or China, or imported into the West as loose herbs and packaged here. A very high standard is usually maintained, although there have been cases of non-authentic herbs being used in pre-packaged remedies. Loose herbs are usually harder to fake or substitute, as they are instantly recognizable by the herbalist. Quite often poor-quality ginseng has been passed off as high-quality. However, you can usually purchase pre-packaged and loose herbs with complete confidence from reputable suppliers in the West.

151

Some herbs will only be supplied on prescription, which you should obtain from your herbalist. Although Chinese herbs are natural they can still be very potent, so great care must be taken with any self-diagnosis or self-treatment. Some of the loose herbs are extremely dangerous poisons. If they are used or prescribed by the herbalist it will be in very small quantities.

Most pre-packaged herbal combinations are sold 'over the counter' and are quite safe. They are usually bought for their effect or for the source illness they treat rather than for conditions alleviated — a practitioner whom you consult as a patient will look, for instance, for stagnating qi or excess damp rather than flu or rheumatism. As such, these remedies may have unfamiliar names or descriptions.

CHINESE PREPARED FORMULAS

The following list is by no means exhaustive, and there are many more combinations available from herbalists. Some combinations may be their own special remedies passed down through generations, while others are very popular and available from any suppliers. The Chinese names are given alongside their English translations (where they have one).

Nourish Yin

Ba Xian Chang Shou Wan   Long Life
Jie Jie Wan   Kai Kit
Liu Wei Di Huang Wan   Six Flavour Tea
Ming Mu Di Huang Wan   Rehmania Tea
Zhi Bai Ba Wei Wan   Eight Flavour Tea

Tonify Yang

Jin Suo Gu Jing Wan   Golden Lock Tea

Tonify Qi

Bu Zhong Yi Qi Wan	Central Ch'i Tea
Liu Jun Zi Pian	Six Gentlemen

Nourish Qi

Dang Gui Pian	Angelica Tea
Dang Gui Su	Tangkuisu

Tonify Both Qi and Blood

Ba Zhen Wan	Women's Precious
Gui Pi Wan	Angelica-Longana Tea
Shuang Bao Su	Panax Ginseng Royal Jelly
Yang Rong Wan	Ginseng Tonic

Expel Wind-Cold

Cang Er San	Xanthium Formula
Chuan Xiong Cha Tiao San	Cindium and Tea Formula
Da Qing Long Tang	Major Blue Dragon Combination
Ge Gen Tang	Pueraria Combination
Gui Zhi Jia Shao Yao Tang	Cinnamon and Peony Combination
Gui Zhi Tang	Cinnamon Combination
Hua Gai San	Ma Huang and Morus Formula
Jing Fang Bai Du San	Schizonepeta and Siler Formula
Jiu Wei Qiang Huo Tang	Chianghuo Combination
Ma Huang Tang	Ma Huang Combination
Ren Shen Bai Du San	Ginseng and Mentha Formula

Shen Su Yin	Ginseng and Perilla Combination
Shi Wei Xiang Ru Yin	Elsholtzia Ten Combination
Xiang Su San	Cyperus and Perilla Formula
Xin Yi San	Magnolia Flower Formula

Expel Wind-Heat

Chai Ge Jie Ji Tang	Bupleurum and Pueraria Combination
Sang Ju Yin	Morus and Crysanthemum Combination
Sheng Ma Ge Gen Tang	Cimicifuga and Pueraria Combination
Yi Qi Cong Ming Tang	Ginseng Astragalus and Pueraria Combination
Yin Qiao San	Lonicera and Forsythia Formula

Flush Downwards

Da Cheng Qi Tang	Major Rhubarb Combination
Fang Feng Tong Sheng San	Siler and Platycodon Formula
Liang Ge San	Forsythia and Rhubarb Formula
Mazi Ren Wan	Apricot Seed and Linun Formula
Run Chang Wan	Linun and Rhubarb Combination
Tiao Wei Cheng Qi Tang	Rhubarb and Mirabilitum Combination
Xiao Cheng Qi Tang	Minor Rhubarb Combination

Subdue Wind

Gou Teng San	Gambir Formula
Wu Yao Shun Qi San	Linderal Formula
Xiao Feng San	Tang-Kuei and Arctium Formula
Xu Ming Tang	Ma Huang and Ginseng Combination
Yi Gan San	Bupleurum Formula

Regulate Qi

Ping Wei Pian	
Xiang Sha Liu Jun Wan	Six Gentlemen + 2

Regulate Blood (Xue)

Fu Fang Dan Shen Pian
Tong Jing Wan
Yun Nan Bai Yao Powder

Expel External Wind

Bi Yan Pian
Gan Mao Ling
Yin Qiao Wan

Clear Heat

Bai Hu Jia Ren Shen Tang	Ginseng and Gypsum Combination
Bai Hu Tang	Gypsum Combination
Bai Tou Weng Tang	Anemone Combination
Chai Hu Qing Gan Tang	Bupleurum and Rehmania Combination

Dao Chi San	Rehmania and Akebia Formula
Huang Lian Jie Du Tang	Coptis and Scute Combination
Huang Qin Tang	Scute and Liquorice Combination
Long Dan Xie Gan Tang	Gentiana Combination
Ma Xing Gan Shi Tang	Ma Huang and Apricot Seed Combination
Qin Jiao Bie Jia San	Chin-Chiu and TS Formula
Qing Shu Yi Qi Tang	Astragalus and Atractylodes Combination
Qing Wei San	Coptis and Rehmannia Combination
Qing Zao Jiu Fei Tang	Eriobotrya and Ophiopogon Combination
San Huang Shi Gao Tang	Gypsum, Coptis and Scutellaria Combination
San Huang Xie Xin Tang	Coptis and Rhubarb Combination
Shao Yao Tang	Peony Combination
Xie Bai San	Morus and Lycium Formula
Yin Chen Hao Tang	Capillaris Combination
Yu Nu Jian	Rehmania and Gypsum Combination
Zhu Ye Shi Gao Tang	Bamboo Leaves and Gypsum Combination

Expel Damp

Ba Zheng San	Dianthus Formula
Bi Xie Fen Qing Yin	Tokoro Combination
Dao Shui Fu Ling Tang	Hoelen and Atractylodes Combination
Du Huo Ji Sheng Tang	Tuhuo and Vaecium Combination

Fang Ji Huang Qi Tang	Stephania and Astragalus Combination
Fen Xiao Tang	Hoelen and Alisma Combination
Huo Xiang Zheng Qi San	Agastache Formula
Liu He Tang	Cardamon Combination
Ma Xing Yi Gan Tang	Ma Huang and Coix Combination
Ping Wei San	Magnolia and Ginger Formula
Wu Lin San	Gardenia and Hoelen Formula
Wu Ling San	Hoelen Five Herbs Formula
Wu Pi Yin	Hoelen and Areca Combination
Yi Yi Ren Tang	Coix Combination
Yin Chen Wu Ling San	Capillaris and Hoelen Formula
Yue Bi Jia Zhu Tang	Atractylodes Combination
Zhu Ling Tang	Polyporus Combination

Resolve Tan (Mucus)

Ban Xia Bai Zhu Tian Ma Tang	Pinellia and Gastrodia Combination
Ding Chuan Tang	Ma Huang and Ginko Combination
Er Chen Tang	Citrus and Pinellia Combination
Su Zi Jiang Qi Tang	Perilla Fruit Combination
Wen Dan Tang	Bamboo and Hoelen Combination
Xiao Qing Long Tang	Minor Blue Dragon Combination

Xing Su San   Apricot Seed and Perilla Combination

Zhi Sou San   Platycodon and Schizonepeta Formula

Subdue Internal Wind

Fu Fang Du Zhong Pian
Jiang Ya Wan

Calm Shen (Spirit)

Chai Hu Jia Long Gu Mu Li Tang   Bupleurium and DP Combination

Gan Mai Da Zao Tang   Liquorice and Jujube Combination

Suan Zao Ren Tang   Ziziphus Combination

Tian Wang Bu Xin Dan   Ginseng and Zizyphus Formula

Yang Xin Tang   Astragalus and Zizyphus Combination

Reduce Food Stagnation

Bao He Wan
Bao Jian Mei Jian Fei Cha   Bojenmi Chinese Tea

Clear Heat and Fire

Long Dan Xie Gan Tang Jiu

Harmonize and Regulate

Chai Hu Shu Gan Tang Jiu
Si Ni San Jiu Xiao Yao San Jiu   Easy Wanderer

Warm the Interior

An Zhong San	Cardamon and Fennel Formula
Da Jian Zhong Tang	Major Zanthoxylum Combination
Dang Gui Si Ni Tang	Tang-Kuei and Jujube Combination
Gan Cao Gan Jiang Tang	Liquorice and Ginger Combination
Hou Po Wen Zhong Tang	Magnolia and Saussurea Combination
Huang Qi Jian Zhong Tang	Astragalus Combination
Li Zhong Tang	Ginseng and Ginger Combination
Wu Mei Wan	Mume Formula
Wu Zhu Yu Tang	Evodia Combination
Xiao Jian Zhong Tang	Minor Cinnamon and Peony Combination

Protect Wei Ch'i

Yu Ping Feng San Jiu	Jade Screen

Tonify Yin

Yi Guan Jian Jiu
Zuo Gui Yin Jiu

Eliminate Dampness

Ping Wei San Jiu
San Miao San Jiu

Eliminate Wind-Damp

Du Huo Ji Sheng Tang Jiu
Juan Bi Tang Jiu

Firm and Gather

Fu Tu Dan
Gui Zhi Jia Long Gu Mu Li
  Tang
Jin Suo Gu Jing Wan
Sang Piao Xiao San

Hoelen and Cuscuta Formula
Cinnamon and DB
Combination
Lotus Stamen Formula
Mantis Formula

HERBAL TINCTURES

The Chinese also use herbal tinctures, which are combinations of up to thirty herbs supplied either as a concentrated extract in an alcohol base or in tablet form. They are usually ordered by name, and are known for the source they treat.

Chinese name	English name	Source treated
Ba Zhen Yi Mu Tang	Women's Precious	Deficient Blood
Bu Zhong Yi Qi Tang	Arouse Vigour	Central Qi
Cai Feng Zhen Zhu	Colourful Phoenix	Heat
Du Huo Ji Sheng Tang	Meridian Circulation	Wind-Cold-Damp
Er Chen Tang	Lucid Clarity	Tan Damp
Gui Pi Tang	Gather Vitality	Spleen Qi-Heart Blood
Gui Zhi Fu Ling Wan	Women's Chamber	Congealed Blood

Chinese name	English name	Source treated
Hu Po Yang Xin Dan	Compassionate Sage	Heart Shen
Liu Wei Di Huang Wan	Quiet Contemplative	Kidney Yin
Liu Jun Zi Tang	Prosperous Farmer	Spleen Qi
Long Dan Xie Gan Tang	Quell Fire	Liver Fire and Damp-Heat
Run Chang Wan	Smooth Response	Dryness
Sha Shen Mai Dong Yin	Wise Judge	Lung Yin and Qi
Shen Tong Zhu Yu Tang	Meridian Passage	Congealed Blood
Tian Wang Bu Xin Dan	Celestial Emperor's Blend	Heart Yin
Tong Yu Jian	Women's Rhythm	Obstructed Qi and Blood
Wen Jing Tang	Women's Journey	Cold & Hot Blood
Wu Ling San	Water's Way	Damp Accumulation
Xiao Yao San	Relaxed Wanderer	Stagnant Liver Qi
Yin Qiao San	Yin Qiao	Wind-Heat
You Gui Wan	Dynamic Warrior	Kidney Yang

By condition or source

Source treated	English name	Chinese name
Central Qi	Arouse Vigour	Bu Zhong Yi Qi Tang
Cold & Hot Blood	Women's Journey	Wen Jing Tang
Congealed Blood	Meridian Passage	Shen Tong Zhu Yu Tang

Chinese name	English name	Source treated
Congealed Blood	Women's Chamber	Gui Zhi Fu Ling Wan
Damp Accumulation	Water's Way	Wu Ling San
Deficient Blood	Women's Precious	Ba Zhen Yi Mu Tang
Deficient Kidney Fire	Temper Fire	Zhi Bai Di Huang Wan
Dryness	Smooth Response	Run Chang Wan
Heart Shen	Compassionate Sage	Hu Po Yang Xin Dan
Heart Yin	Celestial Emperor's Blend	Tian Wang Bu Xin Dan
Heat	Colourful Phoenix	Cai Feng Zhen Zhu
Kidney Yang	Dynamic Warrior	You Gui Wan
Kidney Yin	Quiet Contemplative	Liu Wei Di Huang Wan
Liver Fire & Damp-Heat	Quell Fire	Long Dan Xie Gan Tang
Lung Yin & Qi	Wise Judge	Sha Shen Mai Dong Yin
Obstructed Qi & Blood	Women's Rhythm	Tong Yu Jian
Spleen Qi	Prosperous Farmer	Liu Jun Zi Tang
Spleen Qi – Heart Blood	Gather Vitality	Gui Pi Tang
Stagnant Liver Ch'i	Relaxed Wanderer	Xiao Yao San
Tan Damp	Lucid Clarity	Er Chen Tang
Wind-Cold-Damp	Meridian Circulation	Du Huo Ji Sheng Tang
Wind-Heat	Yin Qiao	Yin Qiao San

These combinations are carefully prepared to exact standards. A typical breakdown (in this case, Dynamic Warrior) looks like this:

Shan Yao	5.1%	Shan Zhu Yu	5.1%
Gou Qi Zi	5.1%	Tu Si Zi	10.3%
Dang Gui	1.7%	Ren Shen	5.1%
Du Zhang	10.3%	Bai Ji Tian	10.3%
Rou Cang Rong	10.3%	Bu Gu Zhi	10.3%
Wu Zhu Yu	2.6%	Wu Wei Zi	5.1%
Niu Xi	6.8%	Shu Di Huang	10.3%

Some of the combinations are no longer known by Chinese names but are all ordered by their Western equivalents; for example, if you wanted a combination to purge the blood you would ask for Purge Blood. The names you can ask for are as follows:

Comfort Shen	Purge Congealed Damp
Consolidate Blood	Purge Damp-Heat
Consolidate Moisture	Purge External Wind
Consolidate Qi	Purge Heat
Disperse Blood	Purge Internal Wind
Disperse Moisture	Purge Moisture
Disperse Qi	Purge Qi
Harmonize Earth and Water	Replenish Essence
Harmonize Fire and Metal	Strengthen Earth
Harmonize Metal and Wood	Strengthen Fire
	Strengthen Metal
Harmonize Water and Fire	Strengthen Water
Harmonize Wood and Earth	Strengthen Wood
Purge Blood	Tonify Blood
Purge Cold	Tonify Moisture
	Tonify Qi

A typical breakdown of ingredients (here, Comfort Shen) would be as follows:

Zhan Zhu Mu	Fu Shen	Long Gu
Ci Shi	Yuan Zhi	Ling Zhi
Ye Jiao Teng	Mai Men Dong	Suan Zao Ren
Chuan Xiong	Hu Po	Wu Wei Zi

Some combination-based herbal prescriptions are ordered by name and source treated:

Name	Source treated
Akebia Moist Heat	Clear Heat and Benefit Damp
Artestatin	Transform Damp
Aspiration	Calm Shen
Backbone	Tonify Yin and Yang
Bupleurum Entangled Qi	Move Qi and Blood
Calm Spirit	Calm Shen
Clear Air	Descend Qi
Clear Heat	Clear Heat
Clearing	Clear Heat and Transform Damp
Coptis Purge Fire	Clear Heat and Drain Fire
Crampbark	Move Blood
Eight Treasures	Tonify Qi and Blood
Enhance	Tonify Qi, Blood, Yin and Yang
Essence Chamber	Benefit Damp
Fertile Garden	Tonify Yin and Blood
Full Force with Astragulus	Tonify Qi
Gastrodia Relieve Wind	Subdue Wind
Ginseng and Gecko	Tonify Qi

Over-the-Counter (Patent) Remedies

Name	Source treated
Heavenly Water	Move Qi
Isatis Cooling	Clear Heat and Cool Blood
Isatis Gold	Release the Exterior
Jin Qian Cao Stone	Clear Heat and Benefit Damp
Minor Blue Dragon	Transform Mucus
Nine Flavour Tea	Tonify Yin
Power Mushrooms	Tonify Qi and Blood
Quiet Digestion	Regulate the Middle
Schizandra Dreams	Calm Shen
Shen Gem	Tonify Qi and Blood
Two Immortals	Regulate the Middle
Unlocking	Move Blood
Women's Balance	Move Qi and Blood
Xanthium Relieve Surface	Release Exterior
Yin Chao Jin	Release the Exterior

A typical breakdown of ingredients (here, Enhance) would be as follows:

Ling Zhi	Da Qing Ye	Bai Lan Gen	Di Ding
Huang Qi	Bai Mu Er	Chuan Xin Lian	Jin Yin Hua
Dan Shen	Ji Xue Tang	Chan Xiang	Yin Yang Huo
Bai Hua She	She Cao	Yu Yin	Rou Cong Rong
Gou Qi Zi	Gan Cao	Wu Wei Zi	Nu Zhen Zi
Bai Shao	He Shou Wu	Kun Bu	Dang Gui
Hu Zhang	Sha Ren	Zi Hua	Chan Pi
Xi Yang Shen	Du Zhong	Bai Zhu	Shu Chi Huang

MUSHROOMS

There are also a number of live culture concentrates that can be purchased. These are dried edible fungi, used singly or in combinations. Traditionally they have been used in China as food supplements to maintain a healthy constitution.

Chinese name	Botanical name
Bai Mo Gu	Grifola frondosus
Bai Mu Er	Tremella fuciformis
Dong Chong Xi Cao	Cordyceps sinensis
Fu Ling	Poria cocos
Ling Zhi	Ganoderma lucidum
Xiang Gu	Lentinus edodes

Combinations

Ling Zhi Cao + Xiang Gu
Ling Zhi Cao + Xiang Gu + Dong Chong Xia Cao
Dong Chong Xia Cao + Bai Mu Er + Ling Zhi Cao + Xiang Gu + Bai Mo Gu

Glossary of Chinese, Botanical and Common Names

PLANTS USED IN CHINESE HERBAL MEDICINE

Plants often have a number of common names and these may vary according to region within the same country. Some Chinese plants, on the other hand, are not generally known in the West and therefore have no common name. The common names given here are intended as a general guide only.

Botanical name	Common name	Chinese name
Acacia catechu	Black cutch	Er Cha
Acanthopanax gracilistylus	–	Wu Jia Pi
Achyranthes bidentata	'Ox knee root'	Niu Xi
Aconite carmichaeli	Prepared root of Szechuan aconite	Fu Zi
Acorus gramineus	Sweet flag	Chang Pu
Adenophora tetraphylla	'Southern sand root'	Nan Sha Shen
Agastache rugosa	Patchouli	Huo Xiang

Botanical name	Common name	Chinese name
Agrimonia pilosa	Agrimony	Xian He Cao
Akebia trifoliata	'Wood with holes'	Mu Tong
Albizzia julibrissin	Mimosa tree bark	He Huan Hua
Alisma orientale	–	Ze Xia
Alisma plantago-aquatica	Water plantain	Ze Xie
Allium savitum	Bulb of garlic	Xie Bai
Allium tuberosum	Seed of Chinese leek	Jiu Zi
Alpinia officinarum	Galangal	Gao Liang Jiang
Alpinia oxyphylla	'Benefit intelligence nut'	Yi Zhi Ren
Amomum cardamomum	Cardamom	Bai Dou Kou
Amomum tsao-ko	'Grains fruit'	Cao Guo
Amomum villosum	Grains of paradise	Sha Ren
Andrographis paniculata	'Thread the heart' lotus	Chuan Xin Lian
Anemarrhena asphodeloides	Anemarrhena	Zhi Mu
Angelica dahurica	Angelica root	Bai Zhi
Angelica pubescens	Angelica root	Du Huo
Angelica sinensis	Chinese angelica	Dang Gui
Aquilaria agallocha	Aloeswood	Chen Xiang
Arca inflata	Cockleshell	Wa Leng Zi
Arctium lappa	Great burdock	Niu Bang Zi
Areca catechu	Betel nut	Da Fu Pi
Arisaema erubescens/ consanguineum	'Jock-in-the-pulpit'	Tian Nan Xing
Arisaema thunbergii	–	Tian Nan Xing

Botanical name	Common name	Chinese name
Aristolochia debilis	Birthwort root	Qing Mu Xiang
Arnebia euchroma	Groomwell herb	Zi Cao
Artemisia annua/apiacea	Wormwood	Qing Hao
Artemisia vulgaris	Common mugwort	Moxa
Asarum sieboldii	Wild ginger	Xi Xin
Asparagus cochinchinensis	Asparagus root	Tian Hen Dong
Aster amellus	Purple aster root	Zi Wan
Aster tataricus	Purple aster root	Zi Wan
Astragalus complanatus	–	Sha Yuan Ji Li
Astragalus membranaceus	Milk vetch root	Huang Qi
Atractylodes chinensis	Atractylodes	Cang Zhu
Atractylodes lancea	Atractylodes	Cang Zhu
Atractylodes macrocephala	Atractylodes	Bai Zhu
Aucklandia lappa	Costus root	Mu Xiang
Belamcanda chinensis	'Arrowshaft'	She Gan
Benincasa hispida	Winter melon	Dong Gua
Biota orientalis	Leafy twig of Arborvitae	Ce Bai Ye
Bletilla striata	Bletilla rhizome	Bai Ji
Bombyx mori	–	Jiang Can
Borago officinalis	Borage	
Boswellia carterii	Frankincense	Ru Xiang
Brucea javanica	'Crow gallbladder seed'	Ya Dan Zi
Bubalus bubalis	Horn of water buffalo	Shui Niu Jiao
Bupleurum chinense	Thorowax	Chai Hu
Caesalpinia sappan	Sappan wood	Su Mu

Botanical name	Common name	Chinese name
Cannabis sativa	Cannabis seeds	Huo Ma Ren
Carthamus tinctorius	Safflower	Hong Hua
Cassia angustifolia	Senna	Fan Xie Ye
Cassia tora	Cassia seeds	Jue Ming Zi
Cephalanoplos segetum	'Small thistle'	Xiao Ji
Chaenomeles speciosa	Japanese quince	Mu Gua
Chrysanthemum indicum	Wild chrysanthemum	Ye Ju Hua
Chrysanthemum morifolium	Chrysanthemum	Ju Hua
Cibotium barometz	Cibot	Gou Ji
Cinnamomum cassia	Cinnamon twigs	Rou Gui
Cirsium japonicum	'Big thistle'	Da Ji
Cistanche deserticolor	Broomrape	Rou Cong Rong
Citrullus vulgaris	Watermelon	Xi Cua
Citrus aurantium	Seville orange	Zhi Shi/Zhi Qiao
Citrus medica v. sacodactylis	Finger citron fruit	Fo Shou
Citrus reticulata	Tangerine peel	Chen Pi/Qing Pi/Ju Luo
Clematis armandii	Clematis	Wei Ling Xian
Clematis chinensis	Clematis	Wei Ling Xian
Cnidium monnieri	'Snakes bed seeds'	She Chuang Zi
Codonopsis pilosula	'Relative root'	Dang Shen
Coix lachrima jobi v. Ma Yuen	—	Yi Yi Ren
Commiphora myrrha	Myrrh	Mo Yao
Coptis chinensis	Golden thread	Huang Lian
Cordyceps sinensis	Mushroom	Dong Chong Xia Cao

Botanical name	Common name	Chinese name
Cornus officinalis	Cornelian cherry	Shan Zhu Yu
Corydalis turtschaninovii	Corydalis	Yan Hu Suo
Corydalis yanhusuo	Corydalis	Yan Hu Suo
Crataegus oxycanthoides	–	Hawthorn
Crataegus pinnatifida	Hawthorn	Shan Zha
Cryptotympana pustulata	Cicada moulting	Chan Tui
Cucumis sativus	Cucumber	Huang Gua
Curcuma aromatica	Tumeric	Chiang Huang
Curcuma longi	Tumeric Rhizome	Jiang Huang
Curcuma phaeocaulis	Zedoary rhizome	E Zhu
Curcuma wenyujin	Tumeric tuber	Yu Jin
Cuscuta chinensis	Dodder seeds	Tu Si Zi
Cuscuta Europaea	Dodder	Tu Si Zi
Cyclina sinensis	Clam shell	Hai Ge kel
Cynanchum atratum	–	Bai Wei
Cynomorium songaricum	'Lock yong'	Suo Yang
Cyperis rotundus	Nutgrass rhizome	Xiang Fu
Dalbergia odorifera	'Descending fragrance'	Jiang Xiang
Daphne genkwa	Daphne flower	Yuan Hua
Daucus alba	White carrot	
Daucus carota	Wild carrot	
Dendrobium spp	Dendrobium	Shi Hu
Dianthus superbus	Pink	Qu Mai
Dichora febrifuga	'Constant mountain'	Chang Shan
Dictamnus albus	Dittany	Bai Xian Pi
Dictamnus dasycarpus	Cortex of Chinese dittany	Bai Xian Pi
Dioscorea batatas	Chinese yam	Bi Xie Xu Duan

Botanical name	Common name	Chinese name
Dioscorea hyperglauca	Fish poison yam rhizome	Bi Xie
Dioscorea opposita	Chinese yam root	Shan Yao
Dipsacus japonica	Japanese teasel root	Xu Duan
Dipsacus silvestus	Teasel	Xu Duan
Dolchos lablab	Hyacinth bean	Bian Dou
Drynaria fortunei	'Mender of shattered bones'	Gu Sui Bu
Eclipta prostrata	Eclipta	Han Lian Cao
Ephedra sinica	Ephedra	Ma Huang
Ephedra vulgaris	Ephedra	Ma Huang
Epimedium brevicornu	Barrenwort	Yin Yang Huo
Epimedium koreanum	Barrenwort	Yin Yang Huo
Epimedium sagittatus	Barrenwort	Yin Yang Huo
Euphoria longan	Flesh of longan fruit	Long Yan Rou
Eriobotrya japonica	Loquat leaf	Pi Pa Ye
Erythrea centaurium	Centaury	
Erythrina variegata	'Bark of the sea panlownia'	Hai Tong Pi
Eucommia ulmoides	Eucommia bark	Du Zhong
Eugenia caryophyllata	Clove flower bud	Ding Xiang
Eupatorium fortunei	Ornamental orchid	Pei Lan
Euphorbia kansui	–	Gan Sui
Euphorbia pekinensis	Peking spurge root	Da Ji
Euryale ferox	–	Qian Shi
Evodia rutaecarpa	Evodia fruit	Wu Zhu Yu
Foeniculum vulgare	Fennel	Xiao Hui Xiang

Glossary

Botanical name	Common name	Chinese name
Forsythia suspensa	Forsythia	Lian Qiao
Fraxinus rhynchophylla	Bark of Korean ash branches	Qin Pi
Fritillaria cirrhosa	Fritillary	Chuan Bei Mu
Fritillaria thunbergii	Fritillary	Zhe Bei Mu
Fritillaria verticillata	Fritillary	Bei Mu
Ganoderma lucidum	Reishi mushroom	Ling Zhi
Gardenia jasminoides	Cape jasmine	Zhi Zi
Gastrodia elata	Gastrodia rhizome	Tian Ma
Gentiana macrophylla	Gentian	Qin Jiao
Gentiana scabra	Chinese gentian root	Long Dan Cao
Ginkgo biloba	Ginkgo	Bai Guo
Glechoma longituba	'Golden money herb'	Jin Qian Cao
Gleditsia sinensis	Chinese honey locust fruit	Zao Jiao Ci
Glehnia littoralis	Root of beech silvertop	Sha Shen
Glycine max	Soyabean	Dan Dou Chi
Glycyrrhiza uralensis/glabra	Liquorice	Gan Cao
Gossampinus malabarica	–	Mu Mian Hua
Grifola frondosus	Mushroom	Bai Mo Gu
Haliotis spp	Abalone shell	Shi Jue Ming
Hedyotis diffusa	'White patterned snake's tongue herb'	Bai Hua She She Cao
Horeum vulgare	Barley sprout	Mai Ya
Houttuynia cordata	'Fishy smelling herb'	Yu Xing Cao
Hyriopsis cumingii	Mother of pearl	Zhen Zhu Mu
Ilex cornuta	Holly	Gou Gou Ye

Botanical name	Common name	Chinese name
Imperata cylindrica	Woolly grass rhizome	Bai Mao Gen
Inula japonica	–	Xuan Fu Hua
Isatis indigotica	Wood root	Ban Lan Gen
Jasminum officinale	Jasmine	Su Xin Hua
Jasminum paniculatum	Jasmine	Su Xin Hua
Juglans regia	Walnut nut	Hu Tao Ren
Juncus effusus	Reed	Deng Xin Cao
Kochia spocaria	Kochia seeds	Di Fu Xi
Laminaria japonica	–	Kun Ru
Ledebouriella sesloides	–	Fang Fen
Lentinus edodes	Mushroom	Xiang Gu
Leonurus heterophyllus	Chinese motherwort	Yi Mu Cao
Leonurus sibiricus	Siberian motherwort	Chong Wei Zi
Lepidium apetalum	–	Ting Li Zi
Ligusticum sinense	Chinese lovage root	Gao Ben
Ligustrum lucidum	Privet fruit	Nu Zhen Zi
Ligustrum wallichii	Szechuan lovage root	Chuan Xiong
Lilium brownii	Lily	Bai He
Lindera strychnifolia	–	Wu Yao
Liquidambar formosana	'All roads open'	Lu Lu Tong
Liriope	Lily turf	Bai He
Litsea cubeba	Aromatic listea root and stem	Don Chi Jiang
Lobelia chinensis	Lobelia	Ban Bian Lian
Lonicera japonica	Honeysuckle flower	Jin Yin Hua
Lonicera parasitica	Honeysuckle	Jin Yin
Lophatherum gracile	Bamboo	Dan Zhu Ye

Botanical name	Common name	Chinese name
Loranthus parasiticus	Mulberry parasite	Sang Ji Sheng
Luffa cylindrica	Loofah	Si Gua Luo
Lycium chinense	Lycium	Crou Qu Zi
Lycopus lucidus v. hirtus	Marsh orchid	Ze Lan
Lycopus virginicus	Bugleweed	
Lygodium japonicum	Climbing fern	Hai Jin Sha Cao
Magnolia biondii	Magnolia	Xin Yi
Magnolia liliflora	Magnolia flower	Xin Yi
Magnolia officinalis	Magnolia bark	Huo Po
Melaphis chinensis	Gall nut of Chinese sumac	Wu Bei Zi
Melia toosendab	Sichuan pagoda tree fruit	Chuan Lian Zi
Mentha arvensis	Mint	Bo He
Mentha piperita	Peppermint	Bo He
Millettia reticulata	Millettia	Chi Hsueh Teng
Morus alba	Mulberry	Sang Ye/Sant Shen Zi/ Sang Zhi
Nauclea rhynchophylla	–	Gou Teng
Nelumbo nucifera	Lotus seed	Lian Zi
Notopterygium incisum	–	Qiang Huo
Ophiopogon japonicus	'Lush winter wheat'	Mai Men Dong
Oroxylum indicum	'Wood butterfly'	Mu Hu Die
Oryza sativa	Rice Sprouts	Dao Ya/Gu Ya
Ostrea spp	Oyster shell	Mu Li
Paennia laciflora/obovata	White peony root	Bai Shao

175

Botanical name	Common name	Chinese name
Paeonia veitchii	Red peony root	Chi Shao
Paeonia suffruticosa	Tree peony	Mu Dan Pi
Panax ginseng	Ginseng	Ren Shen
Panax notoginseng	Pseudoginseng root	San Qi
Panax quinquefolium	American ginseng root	Xi Yang Shen
Patrina villosa	—	Bai Jiang Cao
Perilla acuta	Purple perilla fruit	Su Zi
Perilla frutescens	Perilla leaf	Zi Su Ye
Peucedanum praeruporium	—	Qian Hu
Phellodendron amurense	—	Huang Bai/Huang Bo
Phragmites communis	Common reed	Lu Gen
Phyllostachys nigra	Bamboo shavings	Zhu Ru
Picrorrhiza scohulariiflora	—	Hu Huang Lia
Pinellia ternata	'Half summer'	Ban Xia
Pinus armandii	Pine kernel	Hu Po
Pinus succinifera	Amber	Hu Po
Piper kadsura	'Sea wind vine'	Hai Feng Teng
Piper longum	Long pepper fruit	Bi Bo
Plantago asiatica	Plantain seeds	Che Qian Zi
Plantago depressa	Wild plantain seeds	Che Qian Zi
Plantago paludosa	Plantain	Che Qian
Plantago sibirica	Plantain	Che Qian
Platycodon grandiflorum	Balloon flower	Jie Geng
Polygala sibirica	Milkwort	Yuan Zhi
Polygala tenuifolia	Root of Chinese Senega	Yuan Zhi

Botanical name	Common name	Chinese name
Polygonatum odoratum	Solomon's seal rhizome	Yu Zhu
Polygonum aviculare	Knotweed	Bian Xu
Polygonum bistorta	Bistort	Quan Shen
Polygonum multiflorum	'The vine of Solomon's seal'	Ye Jiao Teng/He Shou Wu
Polyporus umbellatus	Sclerotium	Zhu Ling
Poria cocos	Hoelen	Fu Ling
Portulaca oleracea	Purslane	Ma Chi Xian
Prunella vulgaris	Self-heal	Xia Ku Cao
Prunus amygdalus	Almond	Ba Da Xing Ren
Prunus armeniaca	Apricot kernels	Xing Ren
Prunus consociiflora	Wild cherry	Yu Li Ren
Prunus japonica	Bush cherry pit	Yu Li Ren
Prunus mume	Dark plum	Wu Mei
Prunus persica	Peach kernels	Tao Ren
Pseudostellaria hetrophylla	Lesser ginseng root	Tai Zi Shen
Psoralea corylifolia	Fruit of the scruffy pea	Bu Gu Zhi
Pueraria lobata	Kudzu vine	Ge Gen
Pulsatilla chinensis	Anemone	Bai Tou Eng
Pyrrosia lingua	'Stone reed' leaf	Shi Wei
Raphannus sativus	Radish	Lai Fu Zi
Rehmania glutinosa	Root of Chinese foxglove cooked in wine	Sheng Di
Rehmania glutinosa	Root of Chinese foxglove	Shu Di Huang

Botanical name	Common name	Chinese name
Rheum officinale	Rhubarb	Da Zhang
Rheum palmatum	Rhubarb	Da Huang
Rosa laevigata	Fruit of the Cherokee rose	Jin Ying Zi
Rosa rugosa	Young flower of Chinese rose	Mei Gui Hua
Rubia cordifolia	Madder root	Qian Cao Gen
Rubus chingii	Fruit of Chinese raspberry	Fu Pen Zi
Rubus fruticosus	Blackberry	Fu Pen Zi
Salvia miltiorrhiza	'Scarlet root'	Dan Shen
Sanguisorba officinalis	Burnet-bloodwort root	Di Yu
Santalum album	Sandalwood	Tan Xiang
Sargassum pallidum	Seaweed	Hai Zao
Saussurea lappa	Costus root	Mu Xiang
Schizandra chinensis	Schisandra fruit	Wu Wei Zi
Schizonepeta tenuifolia	–	Jing Jie
Scrophularia ningpoensis	Ningpo figwort	Xuan Shen
Scrophularia nodosa	Figwort	Xuan Shen
Scutellaria baicalensis	Baical skullcap root	Huang Qin
Scutellaria barbata	Skullcap	Ran Zhi Lian
Selaginella doederlenii	'Fir on top of stone'	Shi Shang Bai
Siegesbeckia pubescens	Siegesbeckia	Xi Xian Cao
Sinapis alba	Mustard	Bai Jie Zi
Simlax glabra	Glabrous greenbrier rhizome	Tu Fu Ling
Sophora flavescens	'Bitter root'	Ku Shen

Botanical name	Common name	Chinese name
Sophora japonica	Fruit of the pagoda tree	Huai Jiao
Sophora tonkinensis	'Mountain bean root'	Shan Dou Gen
Sparganium stoloniferum	Bur-reed rhizome	San Leng
Spatholobus suberectus	Millettia root and vine	Ji Xue Teng
Spirodela polyrrhiza	Duckweed	Fu Ping
Stellaria dichotoma	'Silver barbarian kindling'	Yin Chai Hu
Stemona sessilifolia	Stemona	Bai Bu
Stephania tetrandra	–	Fang Ji
Sterculia scaphigera	'Fat big sea' seed	Pang Da Hai
Taraxacum mongolicum	Dandelion	Pu Gong Ying
Taxillus chinensis	'Mulberry parasite'	Sang Ji Sheng
Terminalia chebula	Myrobalon fruit	He Zi
Tetrapanax papyriferus	Rice paper pith	Tong Cao
Tinospora sinensis	'Vine that loosens the sinews'	Kuan Jin Teng
Trachelospermum jasminoides	Star jasmine stem	Luo Shi Teng
Tremella fuciformis	Mushroom	Bai Mu Er
Tribulus terristris	Caltrop fruit	Bai Ji Li
Trichosanthes kirilowii	–	Gua Lou
Triticum aestivium	Wheatsprouts	Fu Xiao Mai
Tussilago farfara	Coltsfoot	Kuan Dong Hua
Typha angustifolia	Cattail pollen	Pu Huang
Typhonium giganteum	'White appendage'	Bai Fu Zi

Botanical name	Common name	Chinese name
Unicaria rhynchophylla	Stems and thorns of Gambir vine	Gou Teng
Vaccaria segetalis	'King who doesn't stay, but departs	Wang Bu Liu Xing
Viola yedoensus	Yedeon's violet	Zi Hua Di Ding
Vitex rotundifolia	Muscadine grape	Man Jing Zi
Xanthium sibiricum	Cocklebur fruit	Cang Er Zi
Zanthoxylum bungeanum	Prickly ash	Hua Jiao
Zanthoxylum piperitum	Japanese prickly ash	Hua Jiao
Zea mays	Cornsilk	Yu Mi Xu
Zingiber officinale	Ginger root	Gan Jiang/ Sheng Jiang
Ziziphus jujuba	Chinese jujube	Da Zao
Ziziphus spinosa	Seed of sour jujube	Suan Zao Ren

OTHER SUBSTANCES USED IN CHINESE HERBAL MEDICINE

Scientific name	Common name	Chinese name
Apis cerano	Honey	Feng Mi
Hydrated calcium sulphate	Gypsum	Shi Gao
–	Brown Sugar	Hong Tang

Useful
Addresses

HERBAL MEDICINE STOCKISTS
(DIRECT AND MAIL ORDER)

In most cities you will find a Chinatown with at least one Chinese herbalist. They are usually more than happy to make up small orders on the spot, but often do not wish to conduct mail order business. For that you will need a herbal importer.

Most countries have herbal importers and, as Chinese herbal medicine increases in popularity, you will find more and more of them. Listed below are a number in the major Western countries. If you write requesting a catalogue or brochure, it is both expedient and courteous to include a stamped addressed envelope.

Inclusion in any listing here is merely a matter of information and in no way implies a recommendation. Similarly, we can also only list the ones we know about: absence from this listing in no way implies any disapproval.

UK

G. Baldwin & Co.
171/173 Walworth Road
London SE17 1RW
Tel: 0171-703 5550

East West Herbs
Langston Priory Mews
Kingham OX7 6UP
Tel: 01608 658862

Neal's Yard Remedies
2 Neal's Yard
Covent Garden
London WC2H 9DP
Tel: 0171–379 0705

Potter's Herbal Supplies Ltd
Leyland Mill Lane
Wigan WN1 2SB
Tel: 01942 234761

Suffolk Herbs
Monks Farm
Pantlings Lane
Kelvedon
Essex C05 9PG
Tel: 01376 572456

USA

East Earth Herbs
PO Box 2082
Eugene
Oregon 97402

Golden Earth Herbs
PO Box 2
Torreon
New Mexico 87061

Institute Herb Company
1190 NE 125th Street, Suite 12
North Miami
Florida 33161
Tel: (305) 899 8704

K'an Herbs
2425 Porter Street, Suite 18
Soquel
California 95073
Tel: (408) 438 9450

North South Herbs
1556 Stockton Street
San Francisco
California 94133
Tel: (415) 421 4907

Tai Sang Trading Company
1018 Stockton Street
San Francisco
California 94108
Tel: (415) 981 5364

Canada

The Herb Works
180 Southgate Drive
Guelph
ON NIG 4P5
Tel: (519) 824 4280

Richter's Herb Specialists
357 Highway 47
Goodwood
ON LOC 1A0
Tel: (905) 640 6677

Australia

Acupuncture Centre
173 Boundary Street
West End
QLD 4101
Tel: (07) 844 2217

Chinese Ginseng Herb
Company
75–77 Ultimo Road
Haymarket
NSW 2000
Tel: (02) 212 4397

Chinese and Herbal Centre
  of Sydney
1st Floor
392–394 Sussex Street
Sydney
NSW 2000
Tel: (02) 261 8863

Yolan Yim
309 Stud Road
Wantirna South
VIC 3152
Tel: (03) 887 0566

New Zealand

Chen's Traditional Chinese
  Herbal Medicine Ltd
107 St Lukes Road
Mt Albert
Auckland
Tel: (09) 849 8239

Chinese Medicine and
  Herbal Clinic
180 Tasman Street
Mt Cook
Wellington
Tel: (04) 384 8232

China Oriental Health
  Centre
Shop 59
Oriental Markets
Britomart Place
Auckland
Tel: (09) 302 3162

Chris Ward and Ziggy Wang
22 Warnock Street
Westmere
Auckland
Tel: (09) 360 2426

Clinic of Traditional
  Chinese Medicine
13 Burgess Road
Johnsonville
Wellington
Tel: (04) 477 0067

Dragonspace
11 Mt Eden Road
Mt Eden
Auckland
Tel: (09) 357 0753

Great Wall Health Centre
21–69 Fanshawe Street
Auckland
Tel: (09) 308 9088

Healthcraft Clinic
11 Rocklands Avenue
Mt Eden
Auckland
Tel: (09) 630 8749

Herbs for Health
146 Hinemoa Street
Birkenhead
Auckland
Tel: (09) 480 2202

Jamu Herbs
Shop 90
Oriental Markets
Birtomart Place
Auckland
Tel: (09) 480 1709
*Manufacturers and distributors
of Indonesian Jamu herbs and
remedies*

Maureen Fleming Natural
    Health Clinic
562 Great South Road
Papatoetoe
Auckland
Tel: (09) 279 3696

Red Beach Natural Therapy
    Centre
17 Red Beach Road
Red Beach
Whangaparaoa
Auckland
Tel: (09) 426 3972

Vicky Martin
40 Titirangi Road
New Lynn
Auckland
Tel: (09) 827 6205

Wah Lee Co Ltd
214–220 Hobson Street
Auckland
Tel: (09) 272 4583

Wong Doo Academy of
    Health
269 Remuera Road
Remuera
Auckland
Tel: (09) 524 2133

Singapore

Chinese Nature Cure
  Institution
BLK 52 Chin Swee Road
#03–33
Singapore 0316
Tel: (65) 532 3962

Sin Chang Cheng
  Traditional Chinese
  Medicine Trading
16 Beach Road
#01–4703
Singapore 0719
Tel: (65) 295 4457

Sinitic Chinese Medicine
  P/L
5001 Beach Road
#04–14
Singapore 0719
Tel: (65) 291 8985

South Africa

Dr Jack Liang
72 Twickenham Avenue
Auckland Park
Johannesburg 2092
Tel: (011) 726 2248

Sui Hing Hong Pty (Ltd)
17 Commissioner Street
Johannesburg 2048
Tel: (011) 838 7704

Dr Kuang
8 Wheatian Buildings
448 Commissioner Street
Fairview
Johannesburg 2048
Tel: (011) 614 1861

COLLEGES, GOVERNING BODIES AND ORGANIZATIONS

As the training and qualifications vary from country to country you are advised to check out your own country's regulations. In the USA the situation even varies from state to state: some allow people to practise with little or no formal qualification, while others require the practitioner to hold a recognized Western medical doctorate. In Europe there is supposed to be standardization via the European Union, but the reality is very different and each country has its own requirements. For example, in the UK there is no legal requirement to hold any qualification, while in France anyone dispensing, prescribing or even doing diagnostic work is, by law, required to hold an orthodox medical doctorate. However, most Chinese practitioners in France set up in business without such a qualification and are never challenged.

You must satisfy yourself about the training and qualifications of your selected practitioner. You should expect to see the qualification written in the language of your own country. Some disreputable practitioners claim to hold qualifications from Chinese medical centres, but when translated into English they merely note the fact that the holder once attended a weekend training seminar on acupuncture or Oriental medicine (one such qualification we have heard of even authorized the holder to sell fish!). You can apply to the various governing bodies for a list of accredited practitioners; usually a small payment is requested. In the UK the Register of Traditional Chinese Medicine is affiliated to the International Register of Oriental Medicine, which was formed in 1975 and issues a Code of Ethics to ensure proper professional relations with patients, fellow practitioners and the public. The International Register of Oriental Medicine monitor their members to make sure that they adhere to the highest standards of sterilization and suitability of premises, and that they are providing the highest levels of competence and practising in a safe, skilful and hygienic manner.

UK

British Herbal Medicine Association
PO Box 304
Bournemouth BH7 6JZ
Tel: 01202 433691

Centre for Complementary Health Studies
University of Exeter
EX4 4PU
Tel: 01392 263263

Council for Acupuncture
179 Gloucester Place
London NW1 6DX
Tel: 0171-724 5330

Council for Complementary
   Medicine
38 Mount Pleasant
London WC1X 0AP

Registry of Chinese
   Medicine
19 Trinity Road
London N2 8JJ
Tel: 0181-883 8431

USA

American Association of
   Acupuncture and Oriental
   Medicine
c/o National Acupuncture
Headquarters
1424 16th Street, NW,
Suite 501
Washington DC 20036
Tel: (202) 332 5794

American Herb Association
PO Box 1673
Nevada City
California 95959

Herb Research Foundation
1007 Pearl Street, Suite 200
Boulder
Colorado 80303
Tel: (303) 449 2265

National Commission for the
   Certification of
   Acupuncturists
c/o National Acupuncture
Headquarters
1424 16th Street, NW,
   Suite 501
Washington DC 20036
Tel: (202) 332 5794

Australia

Acupuncture Ethics and
   Standards Organization
PO Box 84
Merrylands
NSW 2160

Australian College of
   Alternative Medicine
11 Howard Avenue
Mount Waverley
VIC 3149
Tel: (03) 807 4536

Australian College of
   Oriental Medicine
24 Price Road
Lalorama
VIC 3766
Tel: (03) 728 4073

Australian Traditional
 Medicine Society
120 Blaxland Road
Ryde
NSW 2112
Tel: (02) 809 6800

Queensland Institute of
 Natural Science
PO Box 82
Mapleton
QLD 4560
Tel: (074) 429 377

New Zealand

Holistic Health Centre
CPO Box 2273
Auckland
Tel: (09) 307 2588
*Offers training in herbal
medicine remedies, acupuncture,
acupressure and Da Qi*

Singapore

Singapore Chinese
 Physicians Training College
640, Lorong 4 Toa Payoh
Singapore 1231
Tel: (65) 250 3088

Singapore Thong Chai
 Medical Institute
Thong Chai Building
50 Chin Swee Road
#01–00
Singapore 0316
Tel: (65) 733 6905

Example of training and qualification

As the variations between one country and another are so great we can only give you an example of the sort of training and qualification available.

In the UK there is no formal requirement to hold any qualification; nevertheless, excellent training and qualifications are available. The London School of Acupuncture and Traditional Chinese Medicine offers a two-year diploma course in Chinese herbal medicine. Although part-time, the course is very thorough and comprises some 350 hours of classes and a further 200 hours of case study and clinical work. The student's progress is judged through on-course assessment and end-of-year examinations. The course is open to practising acupuncturists who have a grounding in traditional Chinese medicine, Western physiology, pathology and clinical medicine, and at least 200 hours of clinical practice.

The cost, at the time of this book's publication (1995), is £1,500 per year.

The course covers some 250 herbs; their tastes and properties; meridians affected; actions and uses; preparation and dosage, precautions and contra-indications. It also covers some 100 formulae and the study of 50 common conditions, as well as Western pharmacology with its study of the basic constituents in plant medicines. Both case histories and live patients are studied. Students are also required to work on their own, reading classical texts on Chinese herbal medicine and learning about herbs and their properties.

Details are available from:

The Registrar
London School of Acupuncture and Traditional Chinese
  Medicine
60 Bunhill Row
London EC1Y 8QD
Tel: 0171-490 0513

Further Reading

BEINFIELD, Harriet and Efrem Korngold, *Between Heaven and Earth*, Ballantine, 1991

CRAZE, Richard, *Feng Shui for Beginners*, Hodder and Stoughton, 1994

ELLIS, Andrew, Nigel Wiseman and Ken Boss, *Fundamentals of Chinese Acupuncture*, Paradigm Publications, 1989

KAPTCHUK, Ted, *Chinese Medicine: The Web That Has No Weaver*, Congdon and Weed/Rider, 1983

LAN ZHU, Chun, *Clinical Handbook of Chinese Prepared Medicines*, Paradigm Publications, 1989

PORKERT, Manfred, *Essentials of Chinese Diagnostics*, Chinese Medical Publications Ltd, 1983

MABEY, Richard (consultant ed.), *The Complete New Herbal*, Elm Tree Books, 1988

MATSUMOTO, Kikko and Stephen Birch, *Five Elements and Ten Stems*, Paradigm Publications, 1983

MOLE, Peter, *Acupuncture*, Element, 1992

PAHLOW, Manfried, *Healing Plants*, Barron's Educational Series, 1993

ROSS, Jeremy, *Zang Fu*, Churchill Livingstone, 1985

STANWAY, Dr Andrew, *Alternative Medicine*, Bloomsbury Books, 1979

Further Reading

TANG, Stephen and Martin Palmer, *Chinese Herbal Prescriptions*, Rider, 1986

VEITH, Ilza, *The Yellow Emperor's Classic of Internal Medicine*, University of California Press, 1972

YAN CHI, Liu, *The Essential Book of Traditional Chinese Medicine*, Columbia University Press, 1988

YEN HSU, Dr Hong, *How to Treat Yourself with Chinese Herbs*, Keats Publishing, 1993

Index

Index